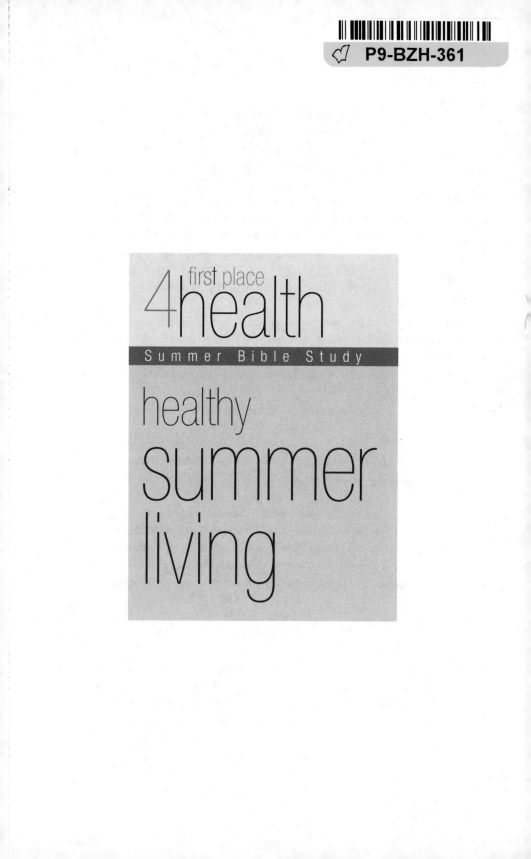

first place
4health
Summer Bible Study

healthy
summer
living

Published by Gospel Light
Ventura, California, U.S.A.
www.gospellight.com
Printed in the U.S.A.

Caution: The information contained in this book is intended to be solely for
informational and educational purposes. It is assumed that the First Place 4 Health
participant will consult a medical or health professional before beginning this or
any other weight-loss or physical fitness program.

Library of Congress Cataloging-in-Publication Data
First Place 4 Health summer Bible study : healthy summer living.
p. cm.
ISBN 978-0-8307-4722-1 (trade paper)
1. Christian women—Prayers and devotions. 2. Bible—Meditations.
3. Summer—Religious aspects—Christianity—Meditations.
4. Christian women—Health and hygiene. I. First Place 4 Health
(Organization) II. Title: First Place for Health summer Bible study.
BV4844.F57 2009
242'.643—dc22
2008054854

Rights for publishing this book outside the U.S.A. or in non-English
languages are administered by Gospel Light Worldwide, an international
not-for-profit ministry. For additional information, please visit
www.glww.org, email info@glww.org, or write to Gospel Light Worldwide,
1957 Eastman Avenue, Ventura, CA 93003, U.S.A.

contents

introduction

But seek first his kingdom and his righteousness,
and all these things will be given to you as well.
MATTHEW 6:33

Summertime can be filled with trips, summer camps and other disruptions in schedules that make it difficult to remain faithful to your commitment to living healthy. *Healthy Summer Living* is a six-week study that was written to provide order to you during the busy summer season without being a burden on your time. It will give you inspiration for each day and also challenge you to stay on course by applying the truths at the core of First Place 4 Health.

You can do this study on your own, or as part of a family devotion time in the home, or in conjunction with a special summer First Place 4 Health group. The Bible study has been created in a five-day format, with the last two days reserved for reflection on the material studied. Keep in mind that the ultimate goal of studying the Bible is not only for knowledge but also for application and a changed life. Don't feel anxious if you can't seem to find the *correct* answer. Many times, the Word will speak differently to different people, depending on where they are in their walk with God and the season of life they are experiencing. If you are doing this study as part of a special summer group, be prepared to discuss with your fellow members what you learned that week through your study.

There are some additional components included with this study that will be helpful as you pursue the goal of giving Christ first place in every area of your life:

- **Group Prayer Request Form:** This form is at the end of each week's study. If you are using this study as part of a group, you can record any special requests that might be given in class.

- **Summertime Helps:** These are valuable tips and suggestions for staying healthy spiritually, mentally, emotionally and physically throughout the summer season.

- **Leader Discussion Guide:** This discussion guide is provided to help the First Place 4 Health leader guide a group through this Bible study. It includes ideas for facilitating a First Place 4 Health class discussion for each week of the Bible study.

- **Two Weeks of Menu Plans with Recipes:** There are 14 days of meals, and all are interchangeable. Each day totals 1,400 to 1,500 calories and includes snacks. Instructions are given for those who need more calories, and recipes for additional summer favorites are included with the menus. An accompanying grocery list includes items that will be needed for each week of meals.

- **First Place 4 Health Member Survey:** If you are using this study as part of a group, fill out this survey and bring it to your first meeting. This information will help your leader know your interests and talents.

- **Personal Weight and Measurement Record:** Use this form to keep a record of your weight loss during the six weeks of the study.

- **Weekly Prayer Partner Forms:** If you are attending a summer session of First Place 4 Health, fill out the weekly prayer partner form and put it into a basket during the meeting. After the meeting, you will draw out a prayer request form, and this will be your prayer partner for the week.

- **Live It Trackers:** The Live It Tracker is for you to complete at home and turn in to your leader at your weekly meetings. If you have a plan, you can remain consistent in practicing the spiritual, mental, emotional and physical disciplines you have begun in First Place 4 Health—even through the summer!

- **Scripture Memory Cards:** These cards have been designed so that you can use them while exercising. It is suggested that you punch a hole in the upper left corner and place the cards on a ring. You may want to take the cards in the car or to work so that you can practice each week's Scripture memory verse throughout the day.

Before you begin your first week of this study, take a moment to write down your goals and strategies for this summer as they pertain to maintaining your spiritual, mental, emotional and physical health.

My goals for this summer are:

Spiritual: _____

_____

_____

_____

_____

Mental: _____

_____

_____

_____

_____

Emotional: _____
_____
_____
_____
_____
_____

Physical: _____
_____
_____
_____
_____

My strategies for reaching those goals are:

Spiritual: _____
_____
_____
_____
_____

Mental: _____
_____
_____
_____
_____
_____

Emotional: _____

_____

_____

_____

_____

_____

Physical: _____

_____

_____

_____

_____

May the next six weeks take you on a joyful journey toward complete wholeness and health! Here's to the journey!

breathing in God's delights

SCRIPTURE MEMORY VERSE
*I delight greatly in the LORD;
my soul rejoices in my God.*
ISAIAH 61:10

Summer is a time for delights. Think of sunny days, picnics in the park, afternoons at the lake and special celebrations with treasured friends and family members.

Our invitation to you during these next six weeks is to give yourself to each wonderful moment of the summer and really drink in all the delights of this special season as you keep your mind, soul, strength and body in balance. Let your ultimate source of delight be found in God. Always keep Him at the center of your life. Let your thoughts rest on Jesus Christ, and let your soul rejoice in all His goodness.

If you are using this study as part of a summer First Place 4 Health group, please complete this week's study before attending the first group meeting. This will allow you to discuss the material with the rest of the group during the discussion time. Also, please complete the Member Survey found on page 165. The information you give on the survey will help your leader tailor the next six weeks to the needs of the whole group.

We'll be spending much of the next six weeks in the book of Proverbs, but we'll also be taking a look at some other passages of Scripture, particularly as we lay the foundation for what's ahead. As you begin this study, take a few moments to read and meditate on the following verses. These passages will describe the foundations of God's work in creating each season—including summer!

According to Genesis 1:14-19, what controls the seasons?

_____

_____

_____

_____

_____

At the end of the fourth day, what did God "see" (see Genesis 1:18)?

_____

_____

_____

_____

In what ways can you honor God by savoring the delights of summer?

_____

_____

_____

_____

What are some of the things you are looking forward to this summer?

_____

_____

_____

_____

What are some of the things that you hope to achieve this summer?

_____

_____

_____

_____

_____

_____

_____

MADE FOR OUR ENJOYMENT

Day 1

Gracious and loving God, thank You for summer and for the special joys You have built into each day. Help me to always delight in You and Your marvelous creation. You are good. Thank You! Amen.

We often think of winter as being a time of cold temperatures and bare branches and summer as a time when the whole earth just seems to burst to life. What kinds of good things might you experience this summer? What delights of creation will you see? What marvels of God's workmanship will you experience? What will you see, smell, hear, taste and touch?

Have you ever stopped to consider the fact that God created much of the earth simply for your enjoyment? He didn't have to make all the vibrant colors that He did. He didn't have to make insects or rocks or leaves or fish with as much intricacy as He did. He didn't have to make waterfalls or rainbows or sunrises or canyons or diamonds.

In Psalm 24:1, King David writes, "The earth is the LORD's, and everything in it, the world, and all who live in it." David learned to delight in the marvels of God's creation and to see the earth and sky as an expression of God's majesty and power. He penned many beautiful passages that express praise to God.

Read Psalm 8:1-9. What exclamation does David use to begin and end this beautiful psalm?

_____

_____

_____

_____

_____

Read Psalm 8:2. In what ways have you seen "children and infants" bringing praises to God?

_____

_____

_____

_____

How might this verse also apply when you consider that we are all God's children (see John 1:12-13)?

_____

_____

_____

_____

How does David describe the heavens in Psalm 8:3? How does this tie in to what you have read in Genesis 1:14-19?

_____

_____

_____

_____

In Psalm 8:4-8, David describes part of mankind's identity and purpose. How would you describe this truth as it relates to your life?

_____

_____

_____

_____

_____

Using the prompts below, name three specific ways that you can rejoice in God's creation and savor the delights of this summer.

God, I thank You for . . .

_____

_____

_____

_____

God, I rejoice in You because . . .

_____

_____

_____

_____

God, I'm so happy that You created . . .

_____

_____

_____

_____

Close your quiet time this day by praising God for the marvels of His wonderful creation!

> *O Lord, my Lord, Your name is majestic in all the earth! Today I will praise You as I meditate on the wonders of Your creation and Your great love for me. Amen.*

Day 2 — DELIGHTS AND CHALLENGES

Lord God, even in the busy days of summer, it is right that I give You thanks and praise. Throughout history, You have dwelt in the praises of Your people. Please come near to me today as I praise Your holy name. Amen.

It is true that summer is a time of delight, but even times of delight can contain some challenges. Think of running a race or learning a new skill—pleasure, work, training, rest and even difficulty are often woven together. Yet Scripture tells us that there is a purpose for everything—absolutely everything. God uses all things, even the challenges we encounter, for His purposes and glory.

King Solomon, the author of Ecclesiastes and much of Proverbs, lets us in on some important secrets about the tapestries God creates. Read Ecclesiastes 3:1-8. What can you learn about the rhythm of God's grace in these verses?

Think through these various times listed in this passage. What are some of the "times" that you are experiencing right now?

_____

_____

_____

_____

_____

Some of the delights and challenges of summer are predictable, while others can catch us by surprise. Think of a few summer activities and events. How are they both a delight and a challenge? (For instance, summertime means having the kids home from school. This can be a delight in that you are able to spend more time with your kids, but it's also a challenge because there's more chaos in the house.)

_____

_____

_____

_____

_____

In 1 Thessalonians 5:18, Paul tells us to "give thanks in all circumstances, for this is God's will for you in Christ Jesus." Focus on one of the times listed in Ecclesiastes 3:1-8 that you've been going through recently. In what ways can you give thanks in all circumstances during this time, even if it is challenging?

_____

_____

_____

_____

Read Ecclesiastes 12:13. How can this verse help you to keep things in perspective as you go through all of life's challenges?

_____

_____

_____

_____

_____

Lord God, You can do all things. Your invitation to me is to take You at Your word and trust in Your goodness, mercy and love. Help me to do that always. Amen.

Day 3 REJOICING ALWAYS

Gracious and loving God, help me to delight in You and the good things You provide for my enjoyment, even when there are difficulties involved. Amen.

As we learned yesterday, we all go through both delightful and challenging times—sometimes at the same time! Often, a challenge can turn into a delight—or perhaps a challenge can be seen as delightful because we can observe God's goodness at work through it. These spiritual seasons are part of the rhythm of God's grace.

The prophet Habakkuk gives us some advice on how to handle things when life becomes more challenging than delightful. Read Habakkuk 3:17-19. What is a recent time in your life when things have felt difficult for you?

_____

_____

_____

_____

In verse 17, Habakkuk lists all that has gone wrong within the nation of Judah. Yet he continues in verse 18 with an incredible truth that we can apply to the challenges we face today. Write Habakkuk 3:18 in the space below, and then spend a few moments meditating on the truth of this verse.

Yet I will _____ _____ _____ _____, I will _____

_____ _____ _____ _____ _____.

What are some specific ways that you can rejoice and also be joyful in the Lord?

_____

_____

_____

_____

_____

_____

Read verse 19. What truths do you learn about God's character in this verse? How might the promises of strength, restoration, and redemption contained in this verse apply to your life today?

_____

_____

_____

_____

_____

_____

O Sovereign Lord, You are the One who controls the seasons of my life. You are my strength and my song. Today I will rejoice in You and Your love, for You are my Savior and my Lord. Amen.

GOD NEVER CHANGES

Lord God, You are the same yesterday, today and forever. Your steadfast love endures throughout the days and seasons and years. Thank You that I can always trust in Your Word. I delight in You. Amen.

Today, we're going to look at several passages of Scripture that describe the unchanging nature of God and the love He has for us. Although spring has just turned into summer and summer will all too soon turn into fall, there is One who never changes. God is always the same. Think about that—the same God who talked with Adam and Eve, Noah, Moses, Abraham, Joseph, Isaiah, Mary and Martha, Paul and a whole host of others throughout history is the same God we worship and serve today. Great joy can be found in that truth as we savor its implications for our lives.

Turn to Hebrews 13:8. Write out this amazing verse in your own words.

_____

_____

_____

_____

_____

Read Jeremiah 31:3. What kind of love does the Lord love you with? How might this knowledge of God's unchanging love apply to your summer activities?

_____

_____

_____

_____

_____

Have you ever stopped to consider the intensity of God's love for you? Throughout the Bible, we are given various pictures of this love. Some simply to show what His love is like, while some give us a greater picture of the depth of this love. For instance, Song of Solomon 8:6 describes an extremely deep love. Read that verse and mediate on its truth, and then complete the sentence below.

God holds me close to His heart. His love for me is stronger than death. God's love for me burns like a blazing fire. When I think about that, I imagine . . .

_____

_____

_____

_____

Part of God's unchanging nature is that His love for us *never changes.* How wonderful is that! David, the psalmist, sang about this incredible unchanging nature of God in Psalm 111. Read this beautiful hymn of praise, and then explain in your own words what David is saying as it applies to your current situation.

_____

_____

_____

_____

Read Malachi 3:6. One of the many benefits of God's unchanging nature is that even if we stray, God's kindness, love and mercy always remain. Of course, the truth of God's grace as found in this verse is not a license for us to sin (see Romans 6:1), but it does provide us with a pledge that even when we falter, He will always love us. Conclude today's study by spend a few moments resting in the knowledge that God's love for you never changes.

> *O Lord God, I will praise You forever and ever. I will extol You with all my heart, for You are deserving of eternal honor and praise. Amen.*

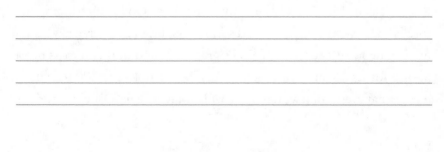

Day 5 THE HEALTH OF WISDOM

Sovereign and loving Lord, Your wisdom is more precious to me than silver and gold. Help me cling to Your wisdom this summer. Your wisdom, like Your word, is eternal. Amen.

If God were to appear to you in a dream tonight and tell you that He would give you whatever you asked for, how would you respond? Be honest. Maybe you would ask for a loved one who is sick right now to be made well. Or maybe you would ask for all the starving children in the world to have enough food. Perhaps your prayer would be simpler than that—maybe you would just ask for enough money to pay your rent this month or that your five-year-old wouldn't drive you crazy.

A new king of Israel was given this opportunity. His father, King David, had just completed a long and successful reign. But when King Solomon took the throne as a young man, he was unsure of the road ahead of him.

Read 1 Kings 3:5-15. Why do you think that King Solomon asked God for wisdom?

_____

_____

_____

_____

_____

Have you ever purposely asked God for wisdom? Why or why not? (If you've never asked God to give you wisdom, why not pause right now and ask God to help you be a person characterized by wisdom.)

_____

_____

_____

_____

_____

_____

Read Proverbs 1:1-7. Describe some of the benefits of wisdom as found in this passage.

_____

_____

_____

_____

_____

_____

Now read Proverbs 1:1-7 again and think of the *opposites* of those words. What might happen if a person *isn't* wise? (For instance, instead of leading a disciplined and prudent life, a person might lead a chaotic and foolish life.) List some of those descriptions below.

_____

_____

_____

_____

_____

_____

Read Proverbs 3:13-18. What are some additional benefits of wisdom?

_____

_____

_____

_____

_____

_____

Read Psalm 111:10. Where does wisdom begin?

_____

_____

_____

_____

Read Psalm 32:8. How might this promise apply to your life?

_____

_____

_____

_____

_____

Read James 1:5. If you are ever lacking wisdom, what does this verse tell you to do?

_____

_____

_____

_____

_____

In what areas of your life do you need wisdom right now? Spend some time today praying that God would give you wisdom and insight in each of these areas in your life.

Gracious God, thank You for being the Author of all wisdom. Thank You for Your promise to guide me and direct me. I look to You. Amen.

REFLECTION AND APPLICATION

Day
6

Merciful Father, You never ask me to do anything without first equipping and preparing me for the task at hand. Thank You for giving me what I need to care for my body, because it is the temple of Your Holy Spirit. Amen.

King Solomon was given the privilege of building an elaborate Temple in which God's people could come and worship Him. The building of this Temple was a labor-intensive project that spanned days, seasons and years. Yet with the coming of Jesus Christ, the "how" and the "where" of worshipping God changed.

Read John 4:21-24. What truth was Jesus telling this woman?

_____

_____

_____

_____

In Acts 7:44-50, we are given additional information about where God dwells today. What is that truth?

_____

_____

_____

_____

The apostle Paul removes all doubt about where God now makes His dwelling place. Read 1 Corinthians 3:16. What incredible truth did you find in that verse?

_____

_____

_____

_____

_____

What are some ways this summer that you can worship God in this new Temple?

_____

_____

_____

_____

_____

End your reflection time today praising God for making your heart His home. Ask God for the continued wisdom you need to care for your body in response to His great love for you.

> *Father, You are my Lord and my God. I praise You today. Thank You that I can worship You in spirit and in truth. Help me to care for my Temple, in which You now make Your home. Amen.*

Day
7

REFLECTION AND APPLICATION

Great and awesome God, You are so good. Thank You for being a God of love. Thank You for loving me so intensely. Thank You for being wise, for always guiding me and for always directing me through the times of my life. I rejoice in You and Your goodness. Amen.

During the course of this past week, we've spent much of our time praising God. We've praised God for His creation. We've praised Him for times of delight and for times when things are challenging. We've praised Him for His unchanging love and because He is the source of all wisdom. Today as we end this first week's study, let's meditate on the first two lines of the Scripture memory verse we've been learning in Isaiah 61:10:

> I delight greatly in the LORD;
> my soul rejoices in my God.

God is so good. As we savor the delights of summer together, let's focus our thoughts right now on His goodness. Let's delight in the Lord and let our soul rejoice in Him.

Creator God, as a bridegroom adorns his head like a priest, or as a bride adorns herself with her jewels, You clothe me in garments of salvation and array me in a robe of righteousness (see Isaiah 61:10). Today I delight greatly in You and my soul rejoices in You, my God.

Group Prayer Requests

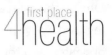

Today's Date: _____

Name	Request

Results

_____

_____

_____

_____

_____

healthy
delights

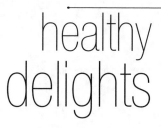

SCRIPTURE MEMORY VERSE
*My soul will rejoice in the LORD
and delight in his salvation.*
PSALM 35:9

Think for a moment about what a perfect summer day would look like for you. Can you see it in your mind's eye? What's the day like? Who's with you? Where are you? What activities are you taking part in (or cheerfully avoiding—like mowing the lawn)? Maybe you envision blue sky, a lazy afternoon in a hammock, or a family get-together around a backyard softball game.

Write down what your day looks like. You may want to use the following prompts:

On my perfect summer's day, I'm . . .

at _____
(location)

with _____
(person or people)

doing _____

_____
(describe what you're doing—or not doing!)

during _____

_____

(favorite time of day)

thinking about _____

_____

wearing my favorite _____

_____

I can smell the scent of _____

_____

and I look forward to_____

_____

Summer gives us a chance to break from our normal routines. Sometimes that's a good thing, as it gives us a chance to stop and take a breather, refocus our priorities and spend more time doing the things that bring us joy. But sometimes a break in routine makes it easier for us to go off course and take a break from the positive disciplines that help keep our life balanced.

How do we keep our balance? It starts with wisdom. From the moment God first granted wisdom to Solomon, the new king began a lifelong quest to discover all the principles of wisdom. First Kings 4:29-34 gives us a glimpse of the inspired work of Solomon. Take a moment to read that passage. How many proverbs did Solomon write? What were some of his other accomplishments?

_____

_____

_____

_____

_____

In the week to come, we're going to take a look at some of the practical applications of wisdom, particularly as those applications relate to this summer for you. Wisdom is always a good thing. It helps you live the life you were truly meant to live. And wisdom always starts with God—He's the Source of all that's wise.

THE BEGINNING OF KNOWLEDGE

Day 1

Gracious God, You are my Father in heaven. I will listen to Your teaching and follow Your instruction, because I know that You love me and know what is best for me. Amen.

In Proverbs 1:7, King Solomon includes a verse that sums up all of the wisdom found in the rest of the book: "The fear of the LORD is the beginning of knowledge, but fools despise wisdom and discipline." As with many of the Proverbs we will be studying in _Healthy Summer Living_, the wisdom in Proverbs 1:7 has two contrasting thoughts. First, knowledge starts with God. _All knowledge._ It doesn't matter who says it or where it's found, God is the author and owner of all the knowledge in the universe. All knowledge ultimately belongs to God. The second thought is that "fools" hate knowledge. What sort of characteristics does a fool have? It might be someone who acts without regard to anyone's wellbeing (including his or her own), or someone who's gullible, or someone who prefers to live in ignorance and darkness.

The encouragement with this proverb, obviously, is to choose the first thought. Through prayer, the power of God and your own choices, you should aim to become a person who chooses knowledge in all you do.

It's easy for people to misinterpret the phrase "fear of the LORD" if they confuse "frightened fear" with "reverent fear." Frightened fear causes people to draw away from God. It causes them to be filled with feelings of guilt, regret and inadequacy instead of overflowing with the joy and hope and confidence that a life centered in Jesus brings. God does not want us to shrink back in fear or run away from Him.

Read Romans 8:1, James 4:8 and I John 4:18. Can you think of a time when you have felt "frightened" fear of God?

In light of those three verses, what does it mean to truly fear the Lord?

A good picture of what it means to fear the Lord is found in Isaiah 6:1-7. Turn to that passage and read Isaiah's experience in the Temple. Let the awe and wonder of this passage fill your soul, and then describe in your own words what happened to Isaiah.

Having a proper fear of the Lord is the key to living a life that pleases God. If you struggle with having frightened fear of the Lord, how might you replace it with reverent fear?

_____

_____

_____

_____

How can a healthy fear of the Lord influence your activities this summer?

_____

_____

_____

_____

God, thank You for the assurance that when I draw near to You, You draw near to me. I have nothing to fear when I am in Your presence. Amen.

LIKE A LOVING PARENT'S VOICE

Day 2

Today, O Lord, I will listen for Your voice. Help me to hear You clearly and respond appropriately. Amen.

Throughout Proverbs, you will often see the phrases "my son" and "my child." Whenever you see these words, realize that the writer is speaking to you as a loving parent would speak to his or her children. It's not meant to sound condescending or as if he is talking down to you. Rather, the tone is one of care and concern. God loves you, and He wants to impart words for wise living to guide you on your path. It's helpful to treat these instructions as God's special message written directly to you. You may even want to substitute your name for the term "my son" or "my child."

Proverbs 1:8-9 is a warning given by a loving father to His beloved child. What is your loving Father asking you to do?

_____

_____

_____

_____

_____

What is the benefit of listening to His instruction?

_____

_____

_____

_____

_____

The following verses in Proverbs all contain a "my son" plea. In the first column, list what your loving Father is asking you to do in that particular proverb. Then, in the next column, write down of the benefit (or benefits) of following His instruction. If you feel comfortable, insert your first name in place of "my son" or "my child."

Proverbs	Instruction	Benefit(s)
Proverbs 3:1-2		
Proverbs 3:21-22		

Proverbs	Instruction	Benefit(s)
Proverbs 4:20-22		
Proverbs 5:1-2		
Proverbs 6:20-22		

Once again, this is quite an impressive list of benefits! Now look back over this list and circle benefits that you would like to have in your life. List them below.

_____

_____

_____

_____

_____

What instructions from your Father in heaven are you asked to follow in order to begin reaping these benefits?

_____

_____

_____

_____

How might any of the instructions you are receiving in your First Place 4 Health group be part of God's instructions to you?

_____

_____

_____

_____

_____

_____

_____

Lord God, You want to shower me with blessings. Help me to live a life worthy of my calling in Christ Jesus so that I can claim all Your promises with bold confidence. Amen.

Day 3 — STRAYING FROM THE DELIGHTS

Gracious and compassionate Father, thank You for giving me personal instruction, straight from the pages of Your Word. Amen.

In the same way that listening to God's instructions will bring health, healing and restoration to your life, ignoring His words will bring unwanted and harmful consequences. In the book of Proverbs, Solomon always presents the loving Father's advice as an earnest plea. However, he doesn't shy away from telling his readers the hard truth of what will happen if they disobey that advice.

Solomon presents this hard truth in creative ways. Some of his descriptions are colorful, or even humorous or whimsical. Studies show there are benefits to this kind of creative teaching. When ideas are presented with action, color and even exaggeration, they tend to stick better in our minds.

Proverbs 6:27-28 is one such whimsical saying that contains great wisdom about the folly of disobedience. Read these verses and summarize what is being taught in the space below.

_____

_____

_____

_____

_____

Not many of us scoop fire into our laps or walk on coals very often, so let's give that whimsical advice some practical applications in everyday terms. Think of a behavior you engaged in recently that did not contribute to life, health or balance. (It could be any behavior that relates to physical, emotional, mental or spiritual balance.) Next, write out your own version of this whimsical proverb using your name, the straying behavior and the probable consequence. The idea here isn't to poke fun at a harmful behavior or the pain that often results, but rather to create a memorable picture that will help you the next time you're tempted in this area. For example:

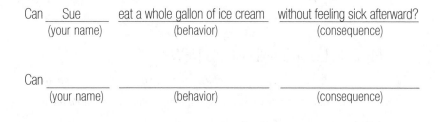

Can ___Sue___ eat a whole gallon of ice cream without feeling sick afterward?
    (your name)   (behavior)   (consequence)

Can _____ _____ _____
    (your name)   (behavior)   (consequence)

Another whimsical example is found in Proverbs 24:30-34. In this passage, Solomon is looking at the life of the sluggard. A sluggard is someone who's lazy, and not in the summer-in-a-hammock kind of way. In this case, Solomon is depicting someone whose life is habitually characterized by a lack of discipline. This person could do something about the chaos in his or her life, but instead does what's easy, even when it's harmful. What lesson can you learn from this passage?

_____

_____

_____

_____

_____

What one step can you take today to turn the predictable consequences of folly into the blessings that come from listening to your Father's voice and obeying His words?

_____

_____

_____

_____

Father, forgive me for the times I do things my way instead of listening to You. Thank You for creative examples of the effects of folly. Help me to observe and learn from what I see. Amen.

Day 4 — CHEERFUL LOOKS AND GOOD NEWS

Lord, just as a loving parent has compassion on a young child, I know that You, O God, understand my weakness and will protect me through the wisdom contained in Your Word. Amen.

Summer can be a time of special joy and health. Often you'll be outside more, breathing clean air, eating fresh produce and enjoying extended times of connection with loved ones. Proverbs 15:30 says, "A cheerful look brings joy to the heart, and good news gives health to the bones."

What might be some everyday examples of "cheerful looks" and "good news" that brings health?

_____

_____

_____

_____

_____

Perhaps the "cheerful look" is your own face in the morning as it is reflected back to you in the mirror. You can choose to either begin the day as a grouch or cheerfully by praising the Lord. Or perhaps the good news that brings health is just that—the healthy number you see on the scale after you've been living a balanced life or the surprised smile your doctor gives you at the end of a checkup.

Read Proverbs 3:5-6. What are the benefits of trusting in the Lord with all your heart and leaning not on your own understanding?

_____

_____

_____

_____

_____

What does Proverbs 3:6 tell you that your path will look like when you trust in the Lord rather than in your own understanding?

_____

_____

_____

_____

_____

What does Proverbs 3:7-8 tell you to do instead of being "wise in your own eyes"?

_____

_____

_____

_____

Think back to what you learned in the last lesson about fearing God. What might a practical example of living out Proverbs 3:7-8 in your life look like?

_____

_____

_____

_____

Thank You, faithful Father, for teaching me the predictable consequences of actions through these wise sayings. Help me to apply this practical wisdom to my life in ways that bring transformation. Amen.

Day 5 — TRUE ABUNDANCE

Lord Jesus, thank You for being a good God. Thank You for inviting me toward health and wholeness. I trust in You. Amen.

Sometimes people think that following God means living a life of drudgery. But nothing could be further from the truth. God invites us to health and wholeness. He offers us abundant life (see John 10:10). Yes, there are challenges to the journey sometimes, but God's way is always best.

When the challenges of life emerge, it's easy to turn to harmful behaviors or substances in an effort to satisfy. But this never provides the true satisfaction we're seeking. We may get a momentary high when eating a dozen jelly donuts, but that's not the path to health, which is what we're really after. The same thing is true for any quadrant of our lives, spiritually, mentally, emotionally or physically. We may want to relax mentally by filling our heads with trashy books, titillating TV or endless pages of Internet drivel. But will that truly bring the mental rest and clarity we need?

God's ways are always best. He offers the real substance of health and wholeness: a life of abundance. When we follow Him, we live the life we were truly meant to live.

Read Proverbs 10:3. How might God's ways and wisdom satisfy your longings instead of harmful behaviors or substances?

_____

_____

_____

_____

_____

_____

Few good things come in life without effort—including health and wholeness. Read Proverbs 12:11. In the context of learning to live a balanced life, what does it mean to "work the land" and have "abundant food"?

_____

_____

_____

_____

_____

For some people, sabotaging their own lives is a familiar practice. They continually make choices that lead to harm and illness. Read Proverbs 14:1. Like the woman mentioned, have you ever found yourself engaging in behaviors that lead to "tearing down your own house"?

_____

_____

_____

_____

_____

Spend some time meditating on the first part of that verse. Pray that God would help you to be wise so that you can continually "build your house"—a good house full of joy, peace, health and freedom. Conclude today's study by praying the words of Proverbs 16:3: "Commit to the LORD whatever you do, and your plans will succeed." When your life is yielded to the Lord, He transforms your desires so that you want what He wants. Commit to the Lord your longings, asking him to bring about the success that leads to life.

> *Lord, You know me better than I know myself. You are in control.*
> *I yield my life to You and Your wisdom. Help me always to delight*
> *in Your goodness. Amen.*

Day
6

REFLECTION AND APPLICATION

Creator God, You have given me this world that You fashioned and
called good as my earthly home. Help me to delight in the wonders of
Your creation, even as I delight in the wonders of You. Amen.

As we have already seen, Proverbs gives us a variety of creative and whimsical examples to help us learn how to avoid the pitfalls of disobedience and live a life of health and wholeness. Yet it also uses examples from God's creation to impart wisdom and knowledge to us. Several of these examples are found in Proverbs 30:24-28. Read each of these Proverbs, and then list what each animal has to teach you.

Proverbs 30:25

_____

_____

_____

_____

_____

Proverbs 30:26

_____

_____

_____

_____

Proverbs 30:27

_____

_____

_____

_____

Proverbs 30:28

_____

_____

_____

_____

Note in verse 26 that the powerless coneys (which are sort of like guinea pigs) build their home in rocky crags, where life is protected and secure. Meditate on the benefits of building your home on the Rock of your salvation (see Matthew 7:24).

> *All of creation sings Your praise, O Lord. Help me to join in the chorus*
> *that is singing praises to You, O God, my Rock and my salvation. Amen.*

Day 7 — REFLECTION AND APPLICATION

Thank You, Lord God, for this day that You have made for my enjoyment. Today I will rejoice in Your love for me. Amen.

Yesterday, we looked at four tiny critters that had big lessons to teach us. Which of these creatures did you identify with or learn the most from? Why?

_____

_____

_____

_____

_____

_____

Today, take a walk outside and spend some time just observing the insects, birds, spiders, reptiles or other animals that are often so easy to overlook. (You might want to incorporate this into your daily walk or take a nature hike apart from your normal exercise routine.) As you walk through God's creation, ask yourself, *What can I learn from a spider? Or that rabbit at the edge of the path? Or that dog that always barks at me when I walk past?* Maybe it will be a bird that has a special message for you! Write down some of your findings in the space on the following page.

_____

_____

_____

_____

_____

_____

_____

_____

_____

Lord, Thank You for wisdom in all places. Today, help me to live a life that is completely devoted to You. You are wise. You are good. Thank You for being You. Amen.

Group Prayer Requests

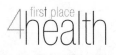

Today's Date: _____

Name	Request

Results

_____

_____

_____

_____

_____

_____

summertime conversations

SCRIPTURE MEMORY VERSE
*A word aptly spoken is like apples of gold
in settings of silver.*
PROVERBS 25:11

Think about the different types of conversations we might have during the summertime. If we have school-age children, we'll probably be talking to our kids more, simply because they're around the house. We might go on vacation during the summer and meet some interesting people on our trip. Maybe we'll strike up a conversation with the person next to us at the pool about a new novel we're devouring or chat to the family at the campsite next to us about what number SPF is best for the day.

Summer can also be a time for family reunions and informal family get-togethers. Maybe we'll run into a great aunt whom we haven't talked with in years or our favorite seafaring uncle who's just blown into town. Or perhaps this summer will simply allow us to have more time to get together for coffee and conversation with trusted and dear friends. Summer allows for different schedules and situations, and enjoying our summertime conversations can be one great way to savor this special season.

This week's memory verse shows us that the conversations we have can greatly influence our experiences of health and wholeness. Like a choice piece or fruit or a finely-crafted piece of jewelry, a good conversation sparkles, gives us joy and creates beauty and light.

The book of Proverbs has a lot to say about our speech. In fact, a running theme throughout Proverbs is that our conversations can be powerful. We have tremendous power to encourage others, speak the truth to them in love, and help guide their lives as we speak wisely about the various situations we have encountered.

In preparation for this week's study, read Proverbs 10:31-32. These verses contain both an exhortation and a warning. As you begin this study, spend some time praying that the Lord would guide you into wise and fitting conversations this summer. Pray that your conversations would always serve to build others up and never tear them down and that they would always reflect the goodness and glory of our Lord and Savior.

Day 1

LISTENING AND SPEAKING

Lord God, how faint the whisper we hear of You, and yet Your voice is full of thunder and power (see Job 26:14). Please give me a listening ear today so that I can hear Your voice through Your Word. Amen.

When you think of God speaking to you, maybe you picture the scene in *The Ten Commandments* where He spoke to Charlton Heston in a deep and booming voice. But if you have ever read the Bible, you have heard God speak. It's as simple as that. God's Word is living and active, and God's Word is God's voice to us. He speaks to us through the pages of Scripture.

God listens to us as well. Any time we pray, we can have confidence that God hears us. Conversation with God is like that. We listen to God as He speaks to us through His Word. We speak to God through prayer. It's a two-way street.

Turn to Ephesians 4:29. As you think about your conversations this week, what are some of the ways that you can put this verse into practice this summer?

_____

_____

_____

_____

_____

James 1:19 has some very practical advice when it comes to having a conversation. What does this verse say, and why might it be hard sometimes to apply this verse?

_____

_____

_____

_____

Do you consider yourself a good listener? Why or why not?

_____

_____

_____

_____

Read Psalm 37:30. In what ways can you live out this verse this summer?

_____

_____

_____

_____

Read Proverbs 15:4. What practical steps can you take this summer to bring healing to people by what you say?

_____

_____

_____

_____

_____

How do you think God speaks to you in healing ways?

_____

_____

_____

_____

Spend some time today praying that God would always guide you in what you say—and what you don't say.

> *Dear Lord, help me to be receptive to words aptly spoken. Help me to season my conversations with Your good salt and always listen to Your voice. Amen.*

Day 2

WISE CONVERSATIONS

O Lord, You are the author of all healthy relationships. Thank You for allowing me to talk with You and to share my life with others. Please guide me in my friendships, and let me be an encourager for Your name's sake. Amen.

When you think about having a "wise" conversation, what comes to mind? Maybe you think about the relationship between a professor and a student, where the learned master imparts wisdom to the pupil. Certainly, wise conversations can happen in that scenario. But wise conversations can also happen between two friends in everyday life. Having a wise conversation simply means that what is said benefits both people in ways that please God. Having wise conversations is part of living a balanced life. Words have power. They can tear down and destroy, but they can also encourage and help to heal.

Read Proverbs 17:27-28. What might it look like to use "words with restraint"?

_____

_____

_____

_____

_____

Have you ever been in a situation where it was wiser to hold your tongue than speak? What was the result?

_____

_____

_____

_____

Proverbs 18:20 contains a creative metaphor: it compares talking to eating. In what ways can a person be "filled" and "satisfied" with wise conversation?

_____

_____

_____

_____

Read Proverbs 25:15. How have you seen this verse put into practice?

_____

_____

_____

_____

Reading Proverbs 26:4 and 5 together almost sounds like a contradiction. In verse 4, the instruction is to "not answer a fool according to his folly, or you will be like him yourself." In verse 5, the instruction is to "answer a fool according to his folly, or he will be wise in his own eyes." Why do you think these verses are arranged side by side like this?

_____

_____

_____

_____

Have you ever found yourself in a situation where both parts of this passage applied? What did you do, or not do?

_____

_____

_____

_____

Read Proverbs 31:26. This verse is often read in context of the entire chapter about the wife of noble character. This particular verse emphasizes how she talks. Give some practical examples of what it means to have "faithful instruction on [your] tongue."

_____

_____

_____

_____

Thank You, loving Father, for wisdom that allows me to savor the delights of summer. Thank You for instruction about wise conversations. Help me always to walk in Your paths. Amen.

WORDS TO WATCH OUT FOR

God, You always speak the truth in love, even when I don't want to hear that truth. Please give me ears to hear and a heart that is open to receive the instruction You want to teach me through today's lesson. Amen.

It can be easy to slip into harmful patterns of conversation, particularly during the summer when we have more time on our hands. In direct contrast to the apt words spoken about in this week's memory verse, Proverbs also gives us instruction about words that are not suitable—no matter what the season or occasion. Living a balanced life means avoiding harmful behaviors. One of the healthy disciplines we can practice this summer is not gossiping, particularly in casual conversations with friends and acquaintances.

Read Proverbs 11:13. What truth is being communicated in this proverb?

Betrayal
no longer trustworthy

What comparison is being made between two different types of people?

What is the difference between betrayal and trustworthiness, according to this verse?

_____

_____

_____

_____

_____

Proverbs 16:28 presents this same truth to us from a slightly different perspective. If a gossip stirs up dissension and separates close friends, by contrast, what does a trustworthy person do (see Proverbs 11:13)?

_____

_____

_____

_____

_____

Proverbs 17:9 and Proverbs 26:20 go into even more depth to this topic. What new ideas are being presented in these verses?

_____

_____

_____

_____

_____

How are trustworthy friendships essential to your health and wholeness?

_____

_____

_____

_____

O Lord, as part of my aim to live a balanced life—the type of life You want me to lead—help me to be a peacemaker, a trustworthy friend, and a person who consistently speaks wise words. Amen.

A CONSTANT ENCOURAGER

Day **4**

Almighty God, thank You for friendships. Help me to be the friend I need to be to others. Thank You for always surrounding me with Your love. Amen.

One of the ways we can help promote health and wholeness in our lives is by encouraging others. When we encourage others, we get a dual blessing: others are blessed by our words, and we also receive a blessing by being an encourager. Simply put, it feels good to build somebody up! It's win-win for everybody involved.

In Romans 1:11-12, Paul writes to the believers in Rome, "I long to see you so that I may impart to you some spiritual gift to make you strong—that is, that you and I may be mutually encouraged by each other's faith." As we begin today's study, spend some time thinking about the power of encouragement, what it feels like to be encouraged, and what a joy it is to bless others when we encourage them.

Read 1 ~~Timothy~~ *Thess*hy 3:2-3. Paul sends a young pastor, Timothy, to the church in Thessalonica to encourage the believers in their faith. The encouragement is especially welcome, because the believers there are going through trials. Think about a time when you were facing a difficulty and someone encouraged you. What was the situation? How did the person encourage you?

_____

_____

_____

the wounds of a friend can be trusted

Think about a time when you gave someone encouragement. What was the result?

_____

_____

_____

_____

_____

_____

Sometimes, we will encourage someone at a time when he or she has strayed or is engaging in behavior that is harmful. At other times, we will need to speak the truth in love to others who have strayed or are engaging in a behavior that is harmful, even though our words may seem like we are wounding them. Read Proverbs 27:6. What is the difference between the profuse (and flattering) words of an enemy and the "wound" of a friend? How is the wound of a friend like a kiss on the lips?

_____

_____

_____

_____

_____

_____

What does Proverbs 27:17 say that reinforces the truth communicated in Proverbs 27:6?

Iron sharpens iron

_____

_____

_____

_____

Complete today's study of encouragement by reading Proverbs 10:32. How does this proverb tie together today's lesson and our memory verse for this week?

_____

_____

_____

_____

_____

Lord God, today I have learned some valuable truths that can help me grow in my relationship with You and others. Help me to apply these truths to my life in meaningful ways. Amen.

AN INCREDIBLE TOOL

Day 5

God, help me to be a person who encourages others and who is able to tell them the truth that they need to hear, even though it may be difficult. Amen.

As we studied yesterday, genuine words of encouragement have the power to strengthen others and build them up. It's one of our essential tools in learning to live a balanced life. Pleasant words come from a heart in tune with God's heart and have a beneficial effect on those saying—and hearing—those words. Proverbs 16:24 says, "Pleasant words are a honeycomb, sweet to the soul and healing to the bones." Let's spend another day thinking through this vitally important subject.

Turn to Proverbs 16:21. What truth does this verse give?

_____

_____

_____

_____

_____

Read Proverbs 16:23. What guides a wise person's words?

_____

_____

_____

_____

_____

List five specific things you can do to continue becoming a person who builds up others by the words that come from your lips.

1. _____

2. _____

3. _____

4. _____

5. _____

End today's lesson by writing a note of encouragement or an email to a friend, or give that person a call. Find a creative and authentic way to let that person know how much God loves him or her.

Father, help me to be an encourager. Let me always speak the truth to others and build them up by the words that come from my lips. Amen.

Day 6 REFLECTION AND APPLICATION

Thank You, Lord God, for giving me practical examples that can help me to more fully grasp the truth of Your Word. Amen.

This week, we have looked at the power of healthy communication. We've seen how we can be effective listeners and how our words have power to help others. We have also seen how true friends build us up by speaking the truth to us in wise and loving ways, and how we can do the same for others.

Who are some of the encouragers in the Bible? When that question is asked, many people mention Barnabas, whose name means "son of encouragement." But there are other encouragers in Scripture. In fact, God directs each of us to encourage one another.

Read 1 Thessalonians 4:18 and 5:14. According to these passages, how are we to encourage others?

_____

_____

_____

_____

_____

Take some time again today to brainstorm some of the ways that you can encourage people this summer. What are some tangible ways that you can show the love of God to others? The more you encourage others, the more this helpful and healing practice will become a regular part of your life.

Spend some time today praying for someone you know who needs encouragement. Let the person know that you are praying for him or her—it will encourage that person to know that you have him or her on your mind and heart. As you close this study, meditate on the words of Galatians 6:9: "Let us not become weary in doing good, for at the proper time we will reap a harvest if we do not give up."

Loving Lord, You are my Lord, and You are my God. I want to live and move and have my being in You! Amen.

REFLECTION AND APPLICATION

My faithful Father, let me always have conversations that are pleasing to You. Help me continually to be the friend I need to be and to have friendships that glorify You. Amen.

Many of the proverbs speak of the value of wisdom and compare lips that speak the truth to a priceless treasure. What is the treasure our memory verse for the week describes?

_____

_____

_____

_____

_____

Turn to Proverbs 20:15. What are "the lips that speak knowledge" compared to in this proverb?

_____

_____

_____

_____

_____

In the space on the following page, or on a separate sheet of paper, draw a treasure chest filled with "priceless jewel" words you can speak to those who are in need of genuine encouragement. As you do, remember that God's Word is always a priceless treasure and that encouraging others with the words of Scripture is always a priceless gift. (You may want to share your treasure chest of valuable words with your small group this week. You can be creative and decorate the page with pictures, glitter, sequins or anything else that helps reinforce the wisdom communicated in Proverbs 20:15.)

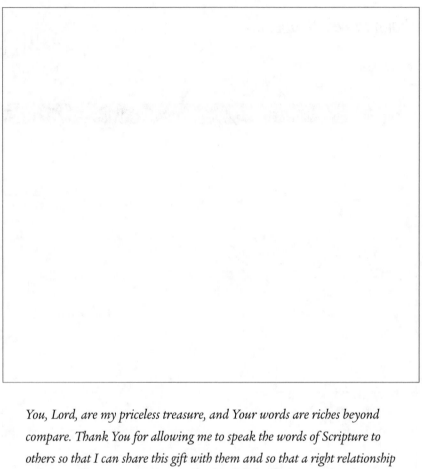

You, Lord, are my priceless treasure, and Your words are riches beyond compare. Thank You for allowing me to speak the words of Scripture to others so that I can share this gift with them and so that a right relationship with You can become their most prized possession as well. Amen.

Group Prayer Requests

4 first place
health

Today's Date: _____

Name	Request

Results

_____

_____

_____

_____

_____

_____

wise choices make summertime delightful

SCRIPTURE MEMORY VERSE
*In the house of the wise are stores of choice food and oil,
but a foolish man devours all he has.*
PROVERBS 21:20

Summer is a time for many wonderful things, but it is also a time when our schedules change. Sometimes this comes as a welcome adjustment, because we get to slow down and take in the experiences of this new season. But at other times our schedules actually ramp up and we have more to do, not less. Unlike many of the other books in the Bible, the book of Proverbs is not arranged according to a particular theme. Instead, the proverbs are often arranged randomly. Inadvertently, this gives us valuable insight into a fundamental truth: Our lives are often a hodgepodge of thoughts and events that consists of many diverse elements that cannot be placed into separate boxes or categories.

In order to live a balanced life, we must have the ability to transition from one aspect of our being to another without losing our footing. The ability to go from one activity to another without losing our balance is a valuable life-skill that we will need to practice during the summer months when we find ourselves juggling all the demands of summer— while trying to enjoy all the pleasures summer brings our way!

What are some of the things you are juggling right now as you strive to keep your balance and focus this summer?

_____

_____

_____

_____

_____

How can the wisdom of living a balanced life be part of both juggling and embracing the delights of summer?

_____

_____

_____

_____

_____

Day 1

A CHOICE FOR THE RIGHT PATH

O Lord God, each day I am faced with so many challenges and choices. How thankful I am that I have chosen to give You first place in my life. When You are my first priority, all the other choices are so much easier for me to make.

Have you ever noticed how our choices play a key role in determining the quality of our lives? For instance, when it's time for a snack, we can choose to eat a handful of fresh strawberries or a carton of cookies. One choice helps promote health and wholeness; the other hinders our success.

Within God's plan and purpose for our lives, there is always the principle of free will. We have the ability to *choose* which path we will take. Certainly, there will be some circumstances in our lives are beyond our control, and at times we may wonder why God has allowed certain things to happen. But we can always be assured that He is *good*. And when faced with a particular situation, we always have a choice as to what our response will be.

Proverbs 4:26 gives us a bit of advice that we can apply to every choice we are asked to make. What is that advice?

_____

_____

_____

_____

_____

With regard to your life, what might a "level path" look like? What elements of moderation and balance allow you to take ways that are firm? In the space below, list two things you can do this summer to make a level path for your feet in each of the following categories:

Physical balance

1. _____

2. _____

Mental balance

1. _____

2. _____

Emotional balance

1. _____

2. _____

Spiritual balance

1. _____

2. _____

Read Proverbs 4:18. What is the path of the righteous compared to in this proverb?

_____
_____
_____
_____
_____

How has your participation in First Place 4 Health allowed your path to grow brighter each day?

_____
_____
_____
_____
_____

Read Proverbs 4:19. In contrast to the growing-ever-brighter path for the righteous described in Proverbs 4:18, how is this path described?

_____
_____
_____
_____
_____

Instead of brightness, we see deep darkness. This path is so dark that the people traveling on it do not even know what makes them stumble! How might the darkness of out-of-control eating be like that dark path?

_____

_____

_____

_____

What specific steps can you take today to ensure that your path grows brighter every day?

_____

_____

_____

_____

Lord, thank You for the gift of free will. Today I choose to use that gift to make wise choices and only take paths that grow brighter each day. Amen.

CHOOSING HEALTHY CHOICES

Day 2

Father, help me to always see my high calling in Christ Jesus and to engage in behavior that leads to healthy consequences. Help me to consider the outcome of my actions and choose what brings glory and honor to You. Amen.

Proverbs often uses illustrations to teach us how to make healthy life choices. One example of this is found in Proverbs 6:6-8, where the writer encourages us to look at ants and learn a lesson from the tiny creatures. In this case, the lesson is directed specifically to those who are lazy or perhaps a bit of procrastinator: "Go to the ant, you sluggard; consider its ways and be wise!" Ants are busy and industrious animals, and the implied instruction is to be like an ant in the sense of taking responsibility for oneself and making correct choices in a season of gathering.

It takes work to plan, shop and prepare wholesome meals. How might driving through the take-out window of a local fast-food restaurant instead of preparing a nutritious meal be similar to the behavior of the sluggard?

_____

_____

_____

_____

_____

Proverbs 6:8 says that the ant stores up food at the harvest. What can you do to support your commitment to health and nutrition that is similar to the behavior of the ant?

_____

_____

_____

_____

_____

Proverbs 6:7 says that the ant "has no _____, no _____ or _____." What lesson in balanced living does this proverb put forth for us?

_____

_____

_____

_____

_____

After using the example of the ant, the writer of Proverbs then asks the sluggard a direct question. Read Proverbs 6:9-11. What is the sluggard—the lazy one—doing in this passage?

_____

_____

_____

_____

Having healthy patterns of sleep is not wrong. In fact, part of living a balanced life is getting the rest we need. So what is unhealthy about the sluggard's sleep patterns? (Hint: What is the end result of the sluggard's choice to fold his hands and take a rest?)

_____

_____

_____

_____

In the context of this passage, what are some potentially harmful results of "folding our hands and resting?"

_____

_____

_____

_____

What is a practical application of "poverty" for us today in the context of living a healthy and balanced life?

_____

_____

_____

_____

Gracious God, help me to never put off until tomorrow what I can do to-day. Help me to always make correct choices that lead to balanced living. Thank You for always loving me. Amen.

Day 3 LAMPS AND LIGHT

Your Word is a lamp to my feet and a light to my path, O Lord (see Psalm 119:105). Today I will shine Your lamp onto all choices I make and let the glory of Your light guide my way. Amen.

It's not fun to think about the potential dangers of summertime, but they do exist. That's why it's important to build in "prudence detectors" to our lives. Accidents can happen, so we need to do things such as wear sunscreen when we are at the beach, watch out for ticks when we are hiking in the forest, avoid eating the potato salad if it's been left out in the sun for too long, and wear a lifejacket whenever we go out in a boat.

The book of Proverbs has a lot to say about living prudently. For instance, Proverbs 22:3 says, "A prudent man sees danger and takes refuge, but the simple keep going and suffer for it." We all encounter warning signs along our way—warning signs that encourage us to pay attention to the path we are taking. Being prudent is simply in our best interest. It allows us to make wise choices whenever danger is near.

Think of a time when you saw a danger that might have sabotaged your ongoing path to health. Perhaps it was an opportunity to go to an all-you-can-eat restaurant or the temptation to watch an old rerun on TV during the time you normally exercise. How did you react to the danger?

What was the result?

_____

_____

_____

_____

_____

_____

Our memory verse this week speaks of having stores of _____ _____ and _____. In this context, it's good to have a pantry stocked with healthy food. Yet this verse also contains a warning. What types of food might entice you to devour all you have?

_____

_____

_____

_____

_____

It's not uncommon to be tempted by a specific type of food—a food that is hard for us to eat in moderation. For instance, maybe your weakness is cookies. If you taste just one cookie, you won't stop until the box is empty! Or perhaps it is potato chips or ice cream. Take a moment to consider the type of food that typically puts you in peril. What specific steps can you take to avoid this food so that you can more fully savor the delights of summer?

don't buy them!
don't start with snacks

_____

_____

_____

It is not just the things we put into our mouth that put us in peril. Proverbs 21:23 warns us of another type of calamity. What is this calamity? How can we avoid it?

_____

_____

_____

_____

How might Proverbs 15:2 give us insight as to how to avoid the pitfalls of foolish words that put us in harm's way?

_____

_____

_____

_____

Rather than having lips that gush folly, Proverbs 15:1 shows us a better way. What is that better way? What are some examples you've seen of this in your own life?

_____

_____

_____

_____

According to Proverbs 15:16, what is better than any form of excess, whether it is food or words? What are some practical examples of how you've seen this verse in action?

_____

_____

_____

_____

Spend some time praising God for who He is and what He has done in your life.

Thank You, Dear God, for giving me a heart overflowing with Your praise rather than filled with excess that leads to destruction. Amen.

HEEDING HEALTHY INSTRUCTION

Day 4

O Lord God, thank You for the wise counsel that's available to me, both from Your Word and from trusted people in my life. Today, I pray for ears that hear and a heart that willingly obeys. Amen.

Sometimes we are tempted to take things easy, even when it comes to healthy disciplines that help keep our lives balanced. It's one thing to take a two-week vacation from work or school, but it's quite another to take a three-month vacation from exercise, reading the Bible, meeting with trusted friends, or healthy eating. The healthy disciplines in our lives are not what make us holy—only Christ can do that—but they can help keep our lives on track. They can help create the climate that produces balanced living and keep our hearts open to all that God intends for our lives.

During an earlier study, we talked about proverbs addressed to "my son" or "my child" and how we can put our name in place of those terms. Turn to Proverbs 19:27 and write it out below, putting in your name wherever "my son" appears.

_____

_____

_____

_____

_____

What does this proverb tell you about the danger of taking a vacation from healthy disciplines—even during the summer months?

_____

_____

_____

_____

What skills do you use that allow you to juggle the changing schedules of summer in a way that better prepares you to enjoy summer's delights? Explain your answer.

_____

_____

_____

_____

Proverbs 28:14 states, "Blessed is the man who always fears the LORD, but he who hardens his heart falls into trouble." How does this verse reinforce the truth found in Proverbs 19:27?

_____

_____

_____

_____

How might doing such things as taking a vacation from attending church, or not participating in First Place 4 Health for a few months, or not attending to the other things that nourish your soul, lead to "hardness of heart"?

_____

_____

_____

_____

What are the results when one allows his or her heart to be hardened?

_____

_____

_____

_____

_____

Read Proverbs 15:32. Who are we really harming when we ignore discipline for a season—that is, when we stop listening to instruction because of our busy schedule?

_____

_____

_____

_____

What insight into living healthily this summer have you gotten from today's lesson?

_____

_____

_____

_____

Although we are prone to think that taking the summer off is being kind to ourselves, what does this verse tell us that we are really doing?

_____

_____

_____

_____

Spend some time praying that the Lord will help you keep on track for the rest of this summer.

> *O Sovereign Lord, You do not take a vacation from caring for me. Help me not to fall into the folly of thinking I can spend my summer away from You and Your words of wisdom that direct my path. Amen.*

Day 5 CHOOSING CONTENTMENT

Mighty God, I thank You for directing my paths and showing me the way that leads to health and holiness of body, mind, heart and soul. Amen.

Our memory verse for the week talks about two types of people: those who are wise and those who are foolish. The wise keep their shelves stocked with nourishing food, but those who lack prudence devour all they have. This verse reinforces the healthy concepts of moderation, self-control and planning for tomorrow instead of only focusing on to-day. These are concepts in learning how to live a healthy and contented life in which we are satisfied with what we have and are not continually giving into our cravings.

Proverbs 30:15 states, "The leech has two daughters. 'Give! Give!' they cry." This verse speaks about those who are not content with what they have. They devour all they have, and then cry out for more. In stark contrast, Proverbs 30:7-9 gives us a lesson on contentment:

> Two things I ask of you, O Lord . . . keep falsehood and lies far from me; give me neither poverty nor riches, but give me only my daily bread. Otherwise, I may have too much and disown you and say, "Who is the Lord?" Or I may become poor and steal, and so dishonor the name of my God.

You may want to spend some time praying this passage to the Lord.

It takes great spiritual maturity to have an abundance of good things and still be dependent on God, the giver of all good gifts! What are some of the dangers of having too much? What are the dangers of having too little? Read Proverbs 30:7-9 again. What two things are Agur, the author of this section of Proverbs, asking of the Lord?

1. _____

2. _____

Based on what Agur is asking for in the rest of this proverb, do you think the deception and lies he wants to be kept from are deception and lies of others? Or is Agur, perhaps, asking that he not be allowed to deceive and lie to himself? Explain your answer.

_____
_____
_____
_____
_____
_____

Can you recall a time when your life was filled with an abundance of good things, but as a result of having this abundance, you neglected your relationship with the Lord? What was the result?

_____
_____
_____
_____
_____

What specific steps do you need to take in order to live contentedly?

_____

_____

_____

_____

> *Lord God, I come to You as a dependent child, asking only for my daily portion of the good things that come from Your loving hands. Thank You for guiding me into all good things. Amen.*

Day 6 — REFLECTION AND APPLICATION

> *Lord, thank You for showing me the pathway to continual healthy living for this summer and beyond. Help me apply the lessons I am learning in a way that will produce results and bring honor and glory to Your name. Amen.*

There are 31 chapters in the book of Proverbs. Some people make it a habit of reading Proverbs through once a month, using the chapter in the book of Proverbs that corresponds with the day of the week as part of their spiritual discipline program.

Today, try this practice for yourself. Whatever day of the month you are doing this lesson on, read the corresponding chapter in Proverbs. As you read, make note of the proverb the Holy Spirit brings to your attention within the chapter. Spend some time meditating on that proverb, distilling the truths the Spirit would have you learn. You might want to write about it in your journal, asking the Lord why He illuminated these specific words of wisdom as you read. End your reflection time by thanking God for being your teacher and for giving you this wonderful textbook of Proverbs as your primer and your guide.

> *Thank You, gracious God, for being my teacher. Thank You for the Holy Spirit's work in my life, and for Jesus, the source of all wisdom. Amen.*

REFLECTION AND APPLICATION

My faithful Father, thank You for calling me into the great family of God and for treating me like a precious, beloved child. Amen.

We have covered a lot of territory during the past four weeks. Much like we do when we come back from vacation, it's time for us to stop and reflect back on the lessons we have learned. We have examined many proverbs and other passages of Scripture and talked about how we can apply these truths to living a healthy and balanced life.

Today, stop and think back over the past four weeks' lessons. If you were sending a postcard to a friend and describing your journey, what one proverb or portion of Scripture would you choose to depict? What one bit of wisdom stands out in your mind as the most valuable lesson you have learned thus far?

_____

_____

_____

_____

_____

_____

After giving this exercise careful thought, find a picture that best describes this lesson. Feel free to sketch your own picture, cut one from a magazine, or download one off of the Internet and print it off. Place your picture on a piece of paper, and write a brief description of the picture on the back. Be prepared to share your Proverbs postcard with your small group the next time you meet.

Lord God, thank You for lessons learned and for loving friends to share these lessons with. Please use my words to help others learn more about the wisdom contained in Your Word. Amen.

Group Prayer Requests

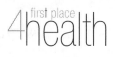

Today's Date: _____

Name	Request

Results

_____

_____

_____

_____

_____

_____

good choices equal healthy results

SCRIPTURE MEMORY VERSE
*A prudent man sees danger and takes refuge,
but the simple keep going and suffer for it.*
PROVERBS 22:3

There are actually three types of wisdom contained in the book of Proverbs: clan wisdom, court wisdom and theological wisdom.

Clan wisdom deals with our interaction with others in our family. When Solomon penned these wise sayings, people often lived together in large extended families, called clans. Often, a household contained an assortment of multi-generation relatives, and towns were sometimes comprised of one big family. Picture a large family reunion—the type that is so often a part of summer—and you'll get a glimpse of what some of the inter-family relationships were like when these proverbs originated. Clan wisdom proverbs teach us how to live in a right relationship with our family, our neighbors and our world. A somewhat humorous example is found in Proverbs 27:14: "If a man loudly blesses his neighbor early in the morning, it will be taken as a curse." If you've ever lived with roommates, in a dormitory, or even with little children who love to watch cartoons early on Saturday morning, you know what this verse is talking about.

Court wisdom deals with our ability to govern with a wise and discerning heart. This type of wisdom has rich application for those of us in leadership roles—whether that be as CEO of a large company or as a parent endeavoring to lead a family down the right path. Court wisdom proverbs also teach us how to relate to those in positions of authority over us, which is a valuable skill in this day and age when it's so easy to just "do our own thing." Proverbs 14:35 is great example of a court wisdom proverb: "A king delights in a wise servant, but a shameful servant incurs his wrath."

The third type of wisdom found in Proverbs, theological wisdom, deals with our relationship with God and the world that He created for our enjoyment. We have looked at a number of these types of proverbs, including Proverbs 1:7, which seems to represent a central theme running throughout the book: "The fear of the Lord is the beginning of knowledge."

Day 1

THE HIGHEST WISDOM

Loving God, You are the source of all wisdom and knowledge. Today I draw near to You, confident that as I do so, You draw near to me. Amen.

Think of all the healthy things you can do in summertime. You can probably be outside more, taking advantage of walks in the park, backyard games with the kids, and bike rides on back lanes. Summertime means enjoying fresh local produce. And summertime often means having more time to reflect on what matters most in your life.

With all the healthy opportunities of summer, what's the single healthiest thing you can ever do? It's to love God. The first and greatest commandment is that you love God with all your heart, all your mind, all your soul and all your strength (see Mark 12:30)! Everything else in your life flows from this.

Let's begin this study by looking at Proverbs 17:3. What wisdom in this verse can help you maintain a right relationship with God?

heat tests metal / the Lord tests our heart

Proverbs 20:27 is a confirmation of this truth. What does this verse say the lamp of the LORD searches?

deep down inside man's heart

How is this searching different from the "testing" described in Proverbs 17:3? Explain the differences between testing and searching as it applies to your motives and attitudes when it comes to living a healthy life.

testing   searching

Read Psalm 139:14 and Matthew 6:33. For some these will be familiar verses, but please read and meditate on them again. How do these verses relate to each other in the context of living a healthy life?

I praise You for how wonderfully You made me. Seek His kingdom first

God created you wonderfully, and He invites you to seek Him first. What are some of the immediate applications of this in your life?

His sight of health

Lord, I praise You because I am fearfully and wonderfully made. You are the one who gives me true wealth, humble honor and an abundant life. Amen.

Day 2

WEALTH, HONOR AND LIFE

Gracious and loving Father, You invite me to be in an intimate love relationship with You. Help me to value this relationship as much as You do and to honor it in the way I live my life before You and others. Amen.

Proverbs 22:4 states that "humility and the fear of the LORD bring wealth and honor and life." At first glance, this might seem strange. The passage seems to imply that the Lord promises that every Christian will always be financially well off, held in high esteem and live a long time. However, we know from other places in Scripture (such as the life of the apostle Paul) and from observations about present-day life that there is a better interpretation to this verse.

The fear of the Lord and righteous living are closely related. Righteous living tends to bring about blessings. So when Proverbs 22:4 states that the fear of the Lord brings wealth, this wealth might be financial in nature, but it can also be spiritual—or a person can be rich in wisdom or in family. When it states that the person will be honored, this might mean that others will hold him or her in high esteem, but it is really God who does the honoring—the person may be unpopular or even scorned by others for doing "the right thing." In the same way, a person who is blessed with "life" may live a long time, but he or she may just live a healthier life—and God may allow that life to be cut short for reasons known only to Him. As Jesus stated in John 10:10, "I have come that [you] may have life, and have it to the full."

Read Proverbs 22:4. What two ingredients are key in producing wealth, honor and life?

respect for the Lord and humility

At first glance, honor and humility seem to be contradictory terms. In what ways can you be humble and still desire and receive honor?

What might wealth, honor and life look like when applied to your health and fitness goals and practices? Think about the application of this verse as it relates to the four quadrants of life: physical, mental, emotional and spiritual.

Wealth:

Honor:

_____

_____

_____

_____

_____

Life:

_____

_____

_____

_____

_____

When you receive wealth and honor and life, to whom does all the praise and honor ultimately belong?

God

_____

_____

_____

_____

_____

The memory verse for this week is Proverbs 22:3. What correlation does this verse have with the truths you just studied in Proverbs 22:4?

_____

_____

_____

_____

_____

How is taking refuge when we see danger part of humility and reverent fear of the Lord?

Knowing and doing what is right gives

How might "keeping on keeping on" in the face of danger be a form of pride in which a person refuses to heed God's warning?

not submitting to Gods teaching, wisdom, guidance.

Is there any area where you are dangerously "keeping on keeping on"? How might continuing in that pathway put your wealth, honor and life in peril?

Write a prayer in your journal asking God for the strength to break any destructive patterns you might have that are keeping you from enjoying the gift of health and wholeness that He longs to give to you.

Gracious and loving Lord, thank You for always loving me. You are the giver of all good gifts. Help me always to live for You. Amen.

THE ONE WHO DIRECTS OUR PATHS

Lord God, as I make plans during these summer months, help me always to take into account the importance of maintaining my relationship with You. Help me to keep You first in all I do—and plan to do! Amen.

When King David wondered what to do, he continually inquired of the Lord (see 1 Samuel 23:2; 30:8, 2 Samuel 5:23). He asked God for wisdom and consulted Him before he made any large-scale plans. David's son Solomon may have picked up that habit from his father, as Proverbs has a lot to say about God and the plans we make.

Begin your study today by looking at the wise words contained in Proverbs 21:30: "There is no wisdom, no insight, no plan that can succeed against the LORD." Continue reading through Proverbs 21:31. What depth of insight does this verse bring to the wisdom contained in Proverbs 21:30?

preparation is important, but seek God's direction; He will always be the victor

What is one of the main battles that those in First Place 4 Health might be engaging in? What are some ways that people who are seeking healthy lifestyles can trust in the Lord to be the source of victory?

temptations

Now look at Proverbs 21:5. What type of diligence do you need to exercise if your plans are going to be profitable?

How might haste, rather than careful planning that includes prayer and consulting God's Word, lead a person into dangerous places? As you ponder this question, remember that danger can take many forms—some veiled and some obvious. *meal planning, out to eat; prep ahead of time for success, not failure. Don't "just do it"*

Proverbs 16:2-4 gives even more insight into this haste-leading-to-poverty problem. Read these verses and then summarize what is being said in your own words. *pray (seek Him first) plan, prepare, with the wisdom and counsel of the Lord. Not doing the 3 will sabotage my healthy eating efforts*

What might "poverty" look like in the context of living a healthy and balanced life?

bankrupt body, sloppy appearance
diabetes, heart attack.

Read Proverbs 16:3 again. Have you ever committed to the Lord your plan to become healthy? If you haven't done so, take some time to do so right now.

> *Gracious God, help me to never step into situations without consulting You first. Help me to always to seek You first in all things, because only as I am willing to seek Your will and way will any good plan succeed. Amen.*

Day 4 RECEIVING FROM THE LORD

> *O Lord, I am Your child. You created me, and You have taught me like a patient parent teaches a child. Thank You for imparting wisdom to me through Your Word. Amen.*

There is something so beautiful about summer mornings. If you get a chance this week, spend a few moments of quiet contemplation outside in the morning. Maybe you will want to take a walk in a nearby park before you head to work. Or maybe you'll simply sit outside on the patio to read your Bible and pray for the day. Whichever you choose, try to listen to the cool of the summer morning. Soak in the stillness and beauty of the day. Spend some time simply thanking God for his creation and His love for you. Meditate on the wonderful truth that God sent His Son to take your sins so that you can have eternal life (see John 3:16), that God loves you (see Jeremiah 31:3), and that He cares for you as a good father cares for his child (see John 1:12).

Begin today's study by reading Proverbs 15:29. God detests wickedness, so He must distance Himself from it. However, He always hears the prayers of the righteous. Knowing what you know about grace (see Ephesians 3:8-9), who is "righteous"?

_____

_____

_____

_____

What comfort does Ephesians 3:8-9 hold for everyone who follows Christ? (Hint: see also 1 Peter 3:12.)

_____

_____

_____

Proverbs 15:24 says, "The path of life leads upward for the wise." What are some practical examples of what this might mean in your life?

_____

_____

_____

_____

Read Proverbs 18:10. How is the name of the Lord like a strong tower to you? In what ways do you run to God?

_____

_____

_____

Sometimes we think of training up our children as more of a challenge than a blessing, but Proverbs presents us with a different truth. In Proverbs 17:6, what does Solomon have to say about the place of children in the family?

Childrens children grandkids are a blessing

What other applications can you draw from this verse when you consider that each of us are all children of God (see 1 John 3:2)?

In Proverbs 23:15-16, Solomon makes a profound statement about his desire for his "son." This may or may not have been Solomon's actual son, but these words were obviously written to a child that Solomon was training up in the ways of wisdom. How does this passage apply when you think of God as your father?

Thank You, Lord, that You are a good God who desires healthy paths for my life. Thank You for loving me and caring for me. Today, I simply receive Your love for me. Amen.

THE CHOICE TO LIVE PEACEFULLY

Loving Lord, You have given me Your Spirit and Your Word so that I can live a life characterized by love, joy and peace. Help me to extend those virtues to all the relationships in my life. Amen.

One of the themes of the book of Proverbs is how it is in our best interest to live at peace with our family and neighbors. In Proverbs 15:15-17, for example, we learn the folly of living in a home characterized by quarrels and strife and how we need to set our priorities straight when it comes to our family relationships. The passage compares a peaceful life to a continual feast—a place of nourishment where there is contentment, worship and an acknowledgement of the love of God. Even though the feast may be a bit on the lean side, it is a place of peace—and that is always better than hatred and strife.

For those of us seeking to live balanced lives, living in homes marked by turmoil and strife can often easily trigger out-of-control eating as we fall into old patterns and use food as a substitute for intimacy and affection. How is this pattern different from the continual feast enjoyed by those with a cheerful heart (see Proverbs 15:15)?

_____

_____

_____

_____

_____

How might having a cheerful heart be an integral part of your endeavors when it comes to moderating your eating?

_____

_____

_____

_____

_____

Take an honest stock of your own life. What is more important in your relationships: a little with fear of the Lord, or great wealth with turmoil (see Proverbs 15:16)? Explain your answer as it applies to having a cheerful heart that enjoys a continual feast.

_____

_____

_____

_____

_____

How might eating a "meal of vegetables" demonstrate more caring to yourself and your family than having a "fattened calf" that produces self-loathing and hatred (see Proverbs 15:17)?

_____

_____

_____

_____

_____

Do you think that Proverbs 15:17 is advocating a vegetarian diet, or do you think that this just a metaphor for a meal that consists more of fruits, whole grains and vegetables than one that consists of large portions of fatty meat?

_____

_____

_____

_____

_____

Proverbs 17:1 reinforces this principle in a slightly different way. What does this verse say is better than a house "full of feasting with strife"?

_____

_____

_____

_____

How might a sensible meal, eaten in peace and quiet, be supportive of your commitment to health and balance?

_____

_____

_____

_____

_____

In Proverbs 21:19, Solomon states this same truth by using a relationship analogy. What do you think Solomon is saying about family relationships in this verse?

_____

_____

_____

_____

Now look at Proverbs 21:9. What does Solomon say is better than living with quarrelsome people?

_____

_____

_____

_____

_____

How might living a life characterized by peace and quiet (especially at mealtime) be a practice you need to incorporate into your endeavor to live a balanced life?

_____

_____

_____

_____

_____

What can you do to make that practice a reality today?

_____

_____

_____

_____

_____

Thank You, gracious and loving Father, for allowing me to see how
turmoil and strife are detrimental to my efforts to live a healthy life.
Help me to find ways to live at peace with You and my family. Amen.

REFLECTION AND APPLICATION

Today, O Lord, I will meditate on Your Word and sing Your praises, for You are the one who showers me with good things that bring delight to my soul. Amen.

In his book *Slaying the Giants in Your Life*, pastor and author David Jeremiah tells of a family in his congregation who took frequent cross-country automobile trips with two small children. Each morning as they set out for the day's journey, the parents would give each child an envelope containing a "treat"—a simple gift and a Scripture passage.

The treat served a dual purpose: the inexpensive gift was something the children could enjoy that day, while the Scripture passage was an eternal-truth passage the family could discuss as they traveled along the road. Each day, the children could look forward to receiving a new envelope—a new surprise and a new Scripture passage. In the same way, as pastor Jeremiah states, "Each new day will bring [us] a new little package from God, with a little grace-gift to refresh us and the always-present truth of God's Word to sustain us."[1]

Many of the proverbs we have studied so far are wonderful verses for parents and children to recite together. Reciting God's Word and then discussing the wisdom contained in those words as a family is a wonderful way of imparting knowledge to those in need of knowledge—while reinforcing the truths in our own hearts. We are all children in the kingdom of God, and many of us need to rerecord the faulty messages that have been erroneously communicated to us in our formative years.

Today, identify one proverb from this week's lesson that you can give to a child within your sphere of influence. Then find an inexpensive gift that complements the lesson that you can give to this child. Finally, if appropriate, plan an outing with that child so that you can discuss the passage together. Enjoy!

*Thank You, loving Father, for practical ideas that reinforce the lessons I
am learning during this study. Thank You for the opportunity to train up
Your children to love and honor You. You are good. Amen.*

Day
7

REFLECTION AND APPLICATION

*Gracious God, You invite me to offer myself as a living sacrifice to You
through the renewing of my mind. Help me today to substitute the mental
thoughts that contradict Your truth with lessons that allow me to use sound
judgment in all my affairs. Amen.*

A few decades back, summer vacations were more arduous than they
are today. Cars were not air-conditioned, station wagons certainly didn't
come equipped with DVD players, and most highways more closely re-
sembled two-lane roads. Meals were usually eaten by the side of the
road from coolers packed before leaving home. Mom carefully guarded
a box of groceries by her feet in the front seat.

Did you ever have one of those family vacations when you were a
child? Sure, you had fun along the way, but it could also be exhausting.
By the time you reached your destination, the provisions in the food
box were dry and stale, and the cooler was anything but cool. Many
families traveled with an unspoken rule that clearly stated, "Thy blad-
der shall be emptied only when the gas tank is empty." As a result,
everyone felt the pressure to not drink much water, even in arid desert
conditions and high temperatures. Short tempers, poor nutrition and
lack of sufficient water often made summer road trips more of an en-
durance test than a vacation.

Part of the process of learning to live in a healthier way is challenging any faulty messages that tell us that taking care of ourselves is not
important—even when we are away from home. We are no longer bound
by any unspoken rules that say time is the only consideration, or a fast-

food meal on the road is the only option, or that our bladders aren't allowed to be full unless the gas tank is empty. Living a balanced life means learning to take care of ourselves at all times, especially when we are on vacation.

If you are planning a family vacation this summer, or have already taken one, what healthy ideas have you incorporated into the trip?

_____

_____

_____

_____

_____

In what ways have you learned to refresh and rejuvenate yourself and your family while on vacation?

_____

_____

_____

_____

Lord, thank You for time to enjoy family. I know that You have created all things for my enjoyment. Help me to care for myself and my family so that I can delight in You and the good things You give me. Amen.

Note

1. David Jeremiah, *Slaying the Giants in Your Life* (Nashville, TN: W Publishing Group, 2001), p. 65.

Group Prayer Requests

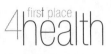

Today's Date: _____

Name	Request

Results

_____

_____

_____

_____

_____

delighting in the Lord

SCRIPTURE MEMORY VERSE
*Whoever gives heed to instruction prospers,
and blessed is he who trusts in the LORD.*
PROVERBS 16:20

During the course of the past five weeks, we have been introduced to the priceless words of wisdom found in the book of Proverbs. As we come to the end of our study, it is important to remember that although Solomon and others in his royal court penned the words of Proverbs, they were inspired, like all Scripture, by God. These proverbs are not meant to be skimmed over quickly, but read slowly and savored. They are genuine food for a tired, hungry soul—a place of refreshment and nourishment on a warm summer day.

Even though your days this summer may be busy and filled with activity, resist the temptation to rush through these proverbs so you can get on to other, seemingly more important, activities. Give yourself time for meditation and application. Write these verses on 3 x 5 cards and carry them with you throughout the day. Review the proverbs you have read in this study often. You might even want to make reading and memorizing some of these wisdom sayings part of your summer travel plans.

Although these proverbs were written down sometime between 971 and 868 B.C., the sage advice they contain is timeless. They can equip you for life in the home, marketplace and workplace. They can give you instructions for living a "wise and prudent" life, no matter what season or situation you find yourself in right now. They can help you keep your feet on the right path—the path that grows brighter every day as you press on toward your health and fitness goals.

As you read and meditate on these proverbs, remember to ask the Holy Spirit—the source of all wisdom—to illuminate the verses He knows you need to apply to your days and years and seasons. This will allow you to live a life that reflects the fear of the Lord, which is truly the foundation of all wisdom.

Day 1 THE LORD GIVES US WISDOM

Gracious and loving Father, thank You for giving me Your Word to guide me down the right path. Thank You for showing me the way and for keeping my feet from turning to the right or to the left. Amen.

Along with the many benefits of wisdom that we have learned about in this Bible study, there also comes a call to responsibility—and action. These proverbs, like all knowledge, only have value in our lives as we put them into practice. Knowledge without application and information without transformation is never our goal in learning to live a healthy life. We are called to be hearers *and* doers of the Word!

Proverbs 2:1-11 gives us a perfect example of the promises contained in Scripture that only become ours to claim when we first take the appropriate action. These action-required-first promises are actually propositional statements. They contain a promise—the "then" of the proposition—that will only become ours when we take the appropriate action—the "if" specified within the statement.

Turn to Proverbs 2:1-4 and read the "if" promises contained in this passage. This is a multifaceted "if" statement containing eight conditions that must be fulfilled before the blessings promised in verses 5, 9 and 11 can be claimed. List the eight "ifs" below. Note that this passage begins with the words "my son," so insert your name in the blank before you begin to list the "ifs." The first one is filled in for you.

_____ , if you:

1. Accept my words _____

2. _____

3. _____

4. _____

5. _____

6. _____

7. _____

8. _____

In Proverbs 2:5, 9 and 11, there are six "thens" that we will reap once we have completed our part of the bargain. List those six benefits below. Once again, the first has been filled in for you.

1. You will understand the fear of the Lord _____

2. _____

3. _____

4. _____

5. _____

6. _____

Now look over your list and circle the benefits you most want to claim as your own by doing the things God calls you to do as a condition of that blessing. Ask God to reveal to you what "if" you need to faithfully fulfill in order for this "then" benefit to become a reality in your life.

> *O Lord, You give wisdom, and from Your mouth comes knowledge and understanding. You hold victory in store for the upright. Help me to do my part so that I can reap Your precious promises. Amen.*

Day 2 KNOWLEDGE OF THE LORD

Lord God Almighty, You are the source of all wisdom. Thank You for sending the Holy Spirit into my heart so that knowledge is pleasant to my soul. Amen.

Yesterday, we studied the if/then propositional statements found in Proverbs 2:1-11. Sprinkled between the "then" statements is some valuable information about the character and attributes of God. Please read Proverbs 2:6-8 again. Just as there were six benefits listed in verses 5, 9, and 11, there are six attributes of God listed in verses 6 to 8. List those attributes in the left hand column of the table below. (We will be completing the right side of the column once we have completed the left side, so leave the right side of the chart blank for now.)

Attributes of God	Benefits of living a healthy life
The Lord gives wisdom	Because the Lord gives me wisdom, I can leave my simple ways behind and renew my mind with His Word.

Attributes of God	Benefits of living a healthy life

For those of us aiming to overcome behaviors that keep us locked in a downward cycle, this list is good news indeed! Now go back and fill in the right hand column of the table by writing down how each attribute of God listed on the left side is beneficial for your efforts in living a balanced life. Conclude your time by writing below a prayer of thanksgiving to God for giving you victory in Christ Jesus.

_____

_____

_____

_____

_____

_____

Thank You, gracious God, for giving me wisdom. You hold victory in store for the upright. You are a shield to those whose walk is blameless, for You guard the course of the just and protect the way of Your faithful ones. Amen.

LIVING IN GOD'S FAVOR

O Lord, because You love me, You allow me to understand what is right and just and fair—every good path. Thank You for guidance and direction and for making my paths straight. Amen.

In Proverbs 3:1-3—yet another passage addressed to "my son"—the wise and loving writer of Proverbs makes a fervent plea to his child. Once again, insert your name at the beginning of this passage, and then fill in the blanks as listed below:

_____ , do not _____ my _____ , but keep my _____ in your _____ , for they will _____ your _____ many _____ and _____ you prosperity. Let _____ and _____ never leave you; _____ them around your _____ , _____ them on the _____ of your heart.

As you read over these words, allow the Holy Spirit to minister to your heart. Are there any commands of the Lord that you struggle with keeping? If so, which ones?

_____

_____

_____

_____

What teaching have you forgotten when it comes to caring for your body, your mind, your heart and your soul in the manner that God intends for you to do?

_____

_____

_____

_____

What are you actively doing to bind God's Word around your neck and write it on the tablet of your heart?

_____

_____

_____

_____

_____

What is the "then" you are promised if you keep the conditions of Proverbs 3:1-3? (Hint: you will find the answer in Proverbs 3:4.)

_____

_____

_____

_____

What does it mean for you to "win the favor and a good name in the sight of God and man"? In other words, what does your life look like when you live in God's favor, and how does that favor impact your efforts to live a healthy life? (Spend some time really thinking through this question. You might want to do your pondering in your journal!)

_____

_____

_____

_____

_____

O Lord, living in Your favor is my heart's desire. Help me to keep Your commandments in my heart and bind them around my neck so that I don't forget what You ask of me. Amen.

Day
4

THE BLESSING OF TRUE RICHES

O Sovereign Lord, I am indeed blessed when I live in the pleasant ways of the peace that only You can give me. Amen.

We ended yesterday's lesson by pondering what it means to have favor in the sight of God and man. Recall some of the things this image brought up for you as you completed yesterday's assignment. Today, Solomon himself gives us a glimpse of the blessings that await those who walk in God's favor.

Begin your reading with Proverbs 3:13-18. In this passage, there are ten benefits listed for the one who "finds wisdom and gains understanding." List those ten benefits below. Because this is also part of the "my son" passage, begin by inserting your name in the blank. Number one and number ten have been filled in for you.

_____, blessed is the [one] who finds wisdom, the [one] who gains understanding, for she [wisdom and understanding] is:

1. More profitable than silver.

2. _____

3. _____

4. _____

5. _____

6. _____

7. _____

8. _____

9. _____

10. Those who lay hold of her will be blessed.

Obviously, not everyone who finds wisdom and gains understanding will be rich in terms of the world's wealth. We don't all get to posses great quantities of gold, silver, rubies and other precious gems. What is really being described in this passage? Think how this might be connected to the acrostic for GRACE: God's Riches At Christ's Expense. Carefully formulate your response in the space below.

_____

_____

_____

_____

_____

_____

_____

_____

Father, wisdom calls out to me so that I can make choices that honor You. Help me to always listen for her voice. I am blessed when I keep Your ways and listen to Your instruction. Amen.

WISDOM'S CALL

Day 5

Thank You, Lord, that wisdom calls out to me from the high places and invites me to seek her. In her hand are riches and honor, and whoever finds her receives favor from the Lord. Help me find wisdom today. Amen.

For the past six weeks, we have traveled through the book of Proverbs on a daily quest for wisdom. Today is the last formal lesson in the *Healthy Summer Living* Bible study, so it is fitting that we learn more about wisdom in order to continue to seek and find her long after summer gives way to fall—and long after we have settled back into our regular autumn routines!

Begin by reading Proverbs 8:2-3. In this passage, wisdom is personified as a woman who calls out to people as they go about their daily routine. Applying this passage to your life, where might you find wisdom today?

_____

_____

_____

_____

_____

Proverbs 8:4-5 reveals who Wisdom is calling out to. Who are the person or persons Wisdom wants to talk to, and why does she want to get their attention?

_____

_____

_____

_____

_____

Now read on through Proverbs 8:6-10. What does Wisdom say about the words she wants to speak in these verses? What motivation does she offer to convince us to listen to her?

_____

_____

_____

_____

_____

_____

Proverbs 8:11 is a reinforcement of the lesson we learned yesterday in Proverbs 3:13-18. According to Proverbs 8:11, what can compare to Wisdom? Elaborate on your response in the space below.

_____

_____

_____

_____

_____

_____

Proverbs 8:12 tells us about the company Wisdom keeps. Whom does she associate with, and why do you think that is so?

_____

_____

_____

_____

_____

_____

Wisdom also tells us what she hates. Look at Proverbs 8:13 and describe what displeases this woman who personifies wisdom. What are some modern-day equivalents of this?

_____

_____

_____

_____

_____

_____

Just as Wisdom hates, she also loves. Proverbs 8:17 tells us what pleases her. Who does she love, and how does she reward those who love her?

_____

_____

_____

_____

_____

Finally, read what Wisdom has to offer those who seek her in Proverbs 8:18-21. How have you seen examples of these benefits in your life?

_____

_____

_____

_____

_____

End your study today by summarizing what you have learned about Wisdom as it applies to your success in learning to live a balanced life. Be sure to include the benefits of wisdom that will help you reach your physical health and fitness goals—as well as the ones that will bring health, healing and balance to you mentally, emotionally and spiritually.

_____

_____

_____

_____

_____

Gracious God, thank You for the wisdom of the proverbs. Thank You for enabling me to apply their wisdom to my life so that I can truly find life and receive favor from You, O Lord, my God. Amen.

REFLECTION AND APPLICATION

Day 6

O Father, You are so good. Whenever I heed Your instructions, I inevitably prosper. Help me to always follow Your pathways. I am so blessed because I trust in You, my Lord and my God. Amen.

During this study, you have been given lots of instruction. You have learned about the benefits of wisdom. You have explored what it means to "fear the Lord." Now, on this day of reflection, the invitation is for you to look back over the lessons of the past six weeks and select five things from this study that have impacted your life. What aspects of the study have been of most benefit to you? What five things have you learned that you have been able to incorporate into your life in meaningful ways? List them below, and then next to each benefit describe how it has made a difference in your life.

1. _____

_____

2. _____

_____

3. _____

_____

4. _____

_____

5. _____

_____

Be prepared to include these five wisdom applications in the testimony you will begin writing tomorrow so that your small group can benefit from the wisdom you have gleaned during this study.

Thank You, sovereign Lord, for placing me on the path that grows brighter every day and for being my companion and my guide on this journey I am making to health, wholeness and balance. Only by Your power and presence can I accomplish the goals I have set as I continue my journey toward health and wholeness. Amen.

Day 7 — REFLECTION AND APPLICATION

Loving Lord, help me to always make prudent choices that reflect my love for You and my desire to grow in grace and knowledge. Amen.

As we have learned during this study, wisdom is a special gift of God. It was given to King Solomon as a result of his request for a wise and discerning heart, and it is given to us by virtue of the Holy Spirit's presence in our lives. In James 1:5, we read, "If any of you lacks wisdom, he should ask God, who gives generously to all without finding fault, and it will be given to him." So today, pray for wisdom, and then allow the Holy Spirit to fill your mind and heart with this special gift.

It is now time to begin preparing your First Place 4 Health testimony by recapping the lessons you have learned—and the progress you have made toward your health and fitness goals—during this six-week session. As you begin to formulate your testimony, be sure to include the delights, challenges, joys and sorrows you have encountered as you studied the book of Proverbs. Talk about any wise words you have discovered that have enabled you to change any destructive behaviors in your life. Then praise God for the new thoughts and attitudes He has given to you that will lead you to health, wholeness and living in God's favor!

As you write your testimony, remember that there will be others in your group who will also want to tell their story, so keep your words precise and focused. Writing them out will help you stay on track as you speak to your group.

Wisdom is indeed a special gift from God. May this gift be yours as you continue your health and wholeness journey!

Loving Father, how thankful I am that You love me. Your wisdom is beyond my intellect and knowledge, yet You willingly give it to me if I seek Your face and listen to Your voice. How blessed I am that You are my God and I am Your beloved child! Amen.

Group Prayer Requests

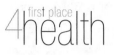

Today's Date: _____

Name	Request

Results

_____

_____

_____

_____

_____

summertime helps

HEALTHY EATING TIPS FOR SUMMER
by Erin DuBroc

Summer can be a blissful time of vacationing, catching up on hobbies and personal projects, or just leisurely enjoying a clear schedule. It can also be a hectic time of traveling cross-country to see family or chauffeuring a van full of kids to sporting events every weekend. However, whether your summer offers you more free time or less, it is important that you work to protect those disciplines you've worked so hard to adopt, such as eating well, being active and growing spiritually. Often summer can be a season when people fall off the proverbial wagon and fail to get back on until New Year's, so it is important that you stay committed to healthy living during this time. Below are some helpful hints about how to keep good nutrition and fitness behaviors stable parts of your routine so that you can enjoy a healthier summer season.

Stay Organized

- If you don't keep healthy foods in your home, chances are you won't make them a part of your diet! Be sure to plan ahead and keep nutritious foods available for yourself and your family.

- When you bring home fresh fruits and vegetables, wash them and then store them in zip-top plastic bags in the fridge. Fruit that is already cut up and ready for use is a lot more appealing than a bunch of whole fruit that has yet to be prepared, so take some time when you get home from the store and make them nibble-ready!

- Maintain some normalcy when it comes to mealtimes. Even with a busy summer schedule, work to keep consistent mealtimes so that you avoid grazing throughout the day, which can easily turn into overeating.

- Keep a limit to how often you eat out each week. It's tempting to eat and run during the summer, but studies show that those who eat out more often tend to eat more and lower quality foods.

- Create a rotating two- to four-week menu that you can use all summer long. Choose some light and cool recipes, create a weekly grocery list, and then enjoy the fact that once you've finished the lists, you won't have to think about what to cook a second longer!

- If you're worried about food spoiling in the fridge while you are on vacation, either buy less at a time, bring the remainder with you on the plane or in the car, or simply buy more frozen vegetables and fruits that will keep for months.

- Set some nutrition-specific goals this summer that will encourage you to eat well and stay on track. Put them on your refrigerator or in a place where you'll often be reminded of them.

Shop Smart

- Healthy eating can actually be easier in the summer, thanks to an abundance of available fresh produce. Start in the produce aisle and stock up on healthy snacks and fresh ingredients for your meals.

- Beware of the junk food aisle. Summer is not an excuse to be lazy and become a junk food addict. If you or your kids are really craving something, buy a small bag and portion it out into zip-top bags when you get home. Remember, these are "seldom" foods that you can enjoy, but you should not be eating them as frequently as "often" foods.

- Try to shop once a week. You buy less that way and ensure that fewer items will spoil. Shopping once a week will also provide you with the freshest foods available, which always taste better.

- Meals at home don't have to be entirely homemade to be nutritious. Many convenience products on the market are a realistic way to save time and energy without compromising quality. For example, pick up a roasted chicken every now and then and make your own vegetable sides at home. Make pizzas with English muffins for a tasty whole grain option. And pick up short-cut ingredients such as frozen meatballs, shredded cheeses and pre-washed and packaged salad greens, fruits and vegetables.

- Check newspaper ads and inserts to take advantage of weekly coupons and specials.

Keep It Fun

- Summer is a great time to involve your kids in food shopping and preparation. Their participation helps to shape positive attitudes about food and gives them feelings of ownership when it comes to the kitchen. This will serve them well later in life!

- Ask your kids to pick three fruits and three vegetables each week. Allow them to choose but always make sure they pick the healthiest versions, such as fresh fruit, frozen fruit or fruit canned in juice as opposed to canned in syrup.

- Have a family fun night where the kids get to plan the meal. Give them some guidelines as far as how many starches and how many vegetables they should choose, but otherwise allow them to make it as wacky as they want.

Stay Safe

- To prevent food-borne illness, it is important to keep cold foods cold and hot foods hot. The former can be especially difficult during these warm summer months.

- When on a picnic, pack food in coolers with freezer packs and set food on the table in dishes sitting on a bed of ice.

- Take groceries straight home from the grocery store—leave the other errands for another day or do them beforehand.

- Wash your hands often and before handling food—especially raw meats, poultry or seafood.

- Avoid cross-contamination by using separate cutting boards for raw meats, poultry or seafood and cooked foods or raw foods like fruits or veggies. Be sure to sanitize kitchen surfaces, cutting boards and utensils thoroughly.

- Use a meat thermometer to check the internal temperature of meat on a grill. Ground meat needs to reach an internal temperature of 160°F, poultry 165°F, and fish and pork 145°F.

Cook and Cool Off Low-Calorie

- When grilling, choose lean cuts of beef, including round, sirloin and loin cuts. Tenderize the meat to increase flavor and texture without adding fat. Marinate them in salsa, low-calorie salad dressing or citrus juices. Grilled chicken breasts, turkey tenders and lamb kabobs also make great alternatives to high-sodium hot dogs and high-fat hamburgers.

- Kick up the health factor by grilling with vegetables and fruits. Make kabobs with fruit and grill them on low heat until the fruit is hot and slightly golden. Serve with a dollop of vanilla yogurt for dessert.

- Water is your best hydrator when temperatures soar, but you can add slices of lemons or strawberries for a light and sweet natural flavor.

- Try a chilled pasta salad made with whole-wheat rotini or macaroni. Search for recipes for light and delicious varieties on sites such as www.cookinglight.com.

- Take advantage of the large variety of in-season fruits and vegetables by getting creative with your salads and chocking them full of all kinds of healthy ingredients. It's a light and cool way to get a lot of your fruit and vegetables in for the day.

- Fruit smoothies are a breeze to make and are a simple way to get your fruit needs for the day. Just toss some fresh or frozen fruit, yogurt and milk in your blender.

- Instead of ice cream, try some frozen 100-percent fruit juice popsicles. Many great flavors are available, such as strawberry, mango, lemon and tangerine!

When On the Road

· Plan ahead! If you're taking a road trip, bring a cooler packed with ice packs and healthy snacks like string cheese, fruit, yogurt, a box of whole wheat crackers, pretzels or baked chips, water and even some sandwiches.

· Depending on how technically savvy you are, you can search for healthy eateries along your route using a GPS system or the Internet. Or you can stop at a visitors center or rest stop and ask the attendants what is nearby.

· If you know that your travels will involve eating out for most meals, it is essential that you not only physically prepare but mentally prepare as well. Make a meal plan as best as you can for each day. If there is a certain food you want to enjoy during your vacation, make allowances for it calorie-wise. In other words, if you plan to splurge a little bit in the evening, go lighter during the rest of the day. Moderation combined with responsibility and common sense will help you to stay on track and still enjoy some treats along the way.

FITNESS TIPS FOR SUMMER
By Vicki Heath

There was a time when the months of June, July and August were called "summer vacation." It was a time when folks played outside until dark. Not any more. Because of busy work schedules, many of us have decided that we do not have time for play. Long walks after dinner have been replaced with our favorite TV program. For most children, active playing has also become a thing of the past. Activities such as riding bikes and running all over the neighborhood have been replaced with television and video games.

Summer is the perfect time to take advantage of the mild temperatures and longer daylight hours and really get out there and do some activities outside. Think back to your childhood for a moment. What was your favorite playground game? Was it jump rope, hopscotch, freeze tag or hide and seek? As you think back to those lazy, hazy, crazy times, try to remember how you enjoyed those active and fitness-filled days of summer. With this in mind, below are some simple playground rules for children and adults.

- **Try Something New.** Summer is the perfect time to take up an activity you've wanted to try. It's a great time for golf lessons, a dance class or even joining a gym. Learning something new will keep your mind fresh and will help to avoid boredom in your fitness routines.

- **Plan a Fitness Vacation.** There are many vacations that involve being very active. Camping, backpacking and hiking are always great choices for family fun. If you vacation in the city, plan a walking tour of historical buildings and parks. Even a day at the zoo can be an opportunity to increase your daily steps. Furthermore, many cruise lines offer a wide variety of fitness opportunities onboard the ship. Wherever you go this summer, make fitness a priority and an appointment every day.

- **Play Every Day.** Make a list of five simple physical activities that you enjoy doing. You might jot down things like taking a walk in the park, mowing the lawn, going for a swim or taking a bike ride. (If you have kids, you might go to the park or school track and take a walk or bike ride after dinner each or every other night—times like those are great opportunities for sharing what's on your heart and making some great memories.) Regardless of what activity you choose, make a date with yourself to do one of these things each day after work so that these activities become an integral part of your life. Then, if you miss your "programmed activity" while you are on a vacation, you will know of other things you can do to stay active.

- **Play in the Water.** Most of us have the opportunity to be near the water at some point during the summer. Water provides the perfect place to safely exercise in the heat and humidity of summer. Swimming is a great cardio workout and is easy on the joints. Don't worry about the fact that the exercise has to be a consistent 30 minutes every day—the minutes will add up as you enjoy your day at the beach, lake or pool. If you are an avid swimmer, consider becoming a certified lifeguard (most community pools and YMCAs offer this certification). Not only would this provide you with a great physical goal to work toward, but it would also enable you to provide a valuable service to your church or community—or even in your own backyard!

- **Go Boating.** Canoeing or any kind of boating activities provides a great overall body workout. (For many of us, just getting into the boat can be quite a challenge!) Many lakes and parks offer rentals and lessons, and if you have never been in a canoe or kayak before, just learning how to do it will be a great workout.

- **Find a Fitness Friend.** Find someone with whom you can do something fun. This could be a family member (you might be surprised how much grandchildren enjoy taking a nature walk!) or even a fellow member in your First Place 4 Health group who shares similar fitness goals. Summer is also a time to make a new fitness friend. You probably know one or two people in your neighborhood who enjoy spending time outside during the evening hours, and they may be interested in joining you in an after-dinner walk.

- **Play Safe and Sensible.** With the nice weather outside, you might be tempted to try and become a champion athlete in just a few days. But it is easy to injure yourself if you are out of shape and push too hard. So start slowly and don't over do it. Practice avoiding the "toos": too much, too soon and too fast. You don't have to do everything full blast! Make that first bike ride for 10 or 15 minutes instead of an hour. Start off with nine holes of golf instead of the full course. If you gradually work your way up to a more challenging workout, you will avoid injuries and most likely stick to it throughout the summer.

- **Prepare Your Fitness Activity in Advance.** When the weather changes, it usually takes 10 days to 2 weeks for your body to get used to the warmer weather. To play it safe, choose higher-intensity activities during cooler morning hours and easier workouts during the heat of the afternoon or evening.

- **Drink the Water.** Staying hydrated is a key element in staying healthy and enjoying the summer. High humidity and high temperatures put demands on the human body, and without the proper hydration, you can quickly run the risk of becoming overheated and dehydrated—even if you are not exercising. If you are outside in the heat, a good rule of thumb is to drink 8 ounces of water every 20 minutes.

Have a healthy, safe and active summer!

Healthy Summer Living
leader discussion guide

Healthy Summer Living is a six-week long Bible study, with one group meeting per week, and is recommended for any member who has completed at least one regular First Place 4 Health session. This shorter session has been specifically designed for First Place 4 Health members who desire to maintain healthy habits during the summer months, when breaks in normal routines can prove challenging to maintaining normal fitness and health routines.

For in-depth information, guidance and helpful tips about leading a successful First Place 4 Health group, spend time studying the *First Place 4 Health Leader's Guide*. In it, you will find valuable answers to most of your questions, as well as personal insights from many First Place 4 Health group leaders.

For the group meetings in this session, be sure to read and consider each week's discussion topics several days before the meeting—some questions and activities require supplies and/or planning to complete. Also, if you are leading a large group, plan to break into smaller groups for discussion and then come together as a large group to share your answers and responses. Make sure to appoint a capable leader for each small group so that discussions stay focused and on track (and be sure each group records their answers!).

Following is a suggested outline for each of the six group meetings.

week one: breathing in God's delights

During this first week, welcome the members to your group and collect the Member Surveys. Begin your Bible study time with a prayer, asking

God to illuminate the heart and mind of each participant.

Take an in-depth look at the creation story in Genesis 1. Outline the seven days and the events that occurred on each day, especially the events of day four, when God created two great lights to control days, years and seasons.

Have the group members think about how they can honor God throughout the seasons. Try going through all of the seasons, identifying the special delights, challenges, joys and sorrows of each.

Take some time for members to discuss in what ways they will rejoice in God's creation this summer. Talk about how delights can be found even in the midst of struggles, how God can turn challenges to delight, and how He can turn sorrows to joy.

Have someone read Habakkuk 3:17-19, then discuss what the prophet is saying and how the members can apply it to their everyday lives.

Write out the two "I will" statements from Habakkuk 3:18. Allow some time for these words to sink in (maybe recite them out loud as a group).

God's steadfast love is part of His character, not a mood dependent on our actions. Talk about that word "steadfast" and what it means as a characteristic of God. Perhaps even take some time to reflect ways in which God has been steadfast in each person's life.

No matter what season we are in—whether it is spiritual or physical, filled with delights or sorrow—don't forget to take time to praise God, for He is good.

week two: healthy delights

Spend some time mulling over wisdom and how it can be important for keeping balance, especially in the midst of the sometimes-unorthodox schedules of summer. Then take a look at Solomon and his wisdom to see why he was qualified to compile the book of Proverbs.

What were the reasons Solomon wrote these proverbs? Read aloud Proverbs 1:2-6 and discuss his purposes for acquiring wisdom and the benefit of studying proverbs.

The fear of the Lord is a difficult phrase for many who confuse "frightened fear" with "reverent fear." Spend some time discussing what "fear of the Lord" means and why it is the beginning of all knowledge.

Sometimes the messages of the Bible can seem distant. Discuss with the group the effects of looking at the proverbs as if they were written to them personally. How would this change the meaning or importance of each verse?

Health and fitness in the world today are often about people's own vain impulses. Ask the participants how God is helping them to shape new ideas and goals for becoming healthier both physically and spiritually.

Solomon uses a variety of ways to impart wisdom. In Proverbs 30, he even uses an assortment of critters. Look at the lessons that each animal has to teach. Discuss why Solomon uses these illustrations and how members can apply this wisdom to their everyday lives.

So much of God's beauty and wisdom is found in nature. Take some time to discuss the nature walk experience and how each individual found wisdom or beauty in creation.

week three: summertime conversations

Read Proverbs 10:31-32 and discuss the practical meanings of this verse. Talk about the big and little things that each person can do to build others up instead of tearing them down.

Take a look at the memory verse for this week. Ask the group what sort of visual imagery the phrase "apples of gold in settings of silver" conjures up. What was the writer's purpose in using this specific simile?

Look at the word "apt" in this week's memory verse and discuss the different meanings of the word. (You might want to even look it up in the dictionary and decide in what way it's used in the proverb.)

It is important for Christians to accept correction with humility and grace. Talk about the difficulties of accepting and giving advice within a Christian community.

It's hard not to listen to those nasty, fun little rumors that grow and spread so easily. Talk for a bit about the harmful effects of gossip, how easy it is to slip into, and some of the ways in which it can be avoided.

On Day 5, the members listed five things they could do to become a person who built others up with their words. Take a moment to share each person's answer to this question.

Have fun decorating and being artistic with your treasure chest drawing from Day 7. Don't be afraid to share with the group what you've created, and take some time to look at their creations.

Close the study time with a word of prayer, asking God to show each member what it means to be rich in His eyes.

week four: wise choices make summertime delightful

At times the book of Proverbs can feel random, but that random arrangement can impart wisdom to those managing busy lives. Discuss some of the things members are juggling as they strive to keep their balance and focus this summer. How can the wisdom of living a balanced life be part of both juggling and embracing the delights of summer?

Proverbs 4:26 gives sound advice that can be applied to every choice the members are asked to make. Discuss what that advice is and what "a level path" might look like in their lives.

Discuss what elements of moderation allow participants to take ways that are firm. Talk about this question as it pertains to each quadrant of a balanced life: physically, mentally, spiritually and emotionally.

Discuss the balance between overworking and becoming like the sluggard in Proverbs 6:9-11. In what ways can members avoid driving themselves too hard without slipping into lazy habits?

After reading about the sluggard, talk about some of the ways people become "lazy"—especially as it pertains to exercise and eating healthy.

Summer can be a much-needed vacation for both body and soul. But there are dangers in taking a three-month leave of absence from healthy living. Discuss the consequences of taking a break from exercising one's mind, body and soul. In what ways can the members stay diligent?

Take a look at Agur's words in the proverbs from Day 5. Discuss the pitfalls of having too much and the dangers of having too little.

Ask participants the specific steps they need to take in order to live a contented life. Have them explain their answers.

On Day 7, group members were instructed to create a picture postcard about the most valuable lesson they had learned thus far in the *Healthy Summer Living* study. Have each person share their cards.

week five: good choices equal healthy results

Take a look at the three types of wisdom in Proverbs: clan wisdom, court wisdom and theological wisdom. Discuss what each type of wisdom has to offer those in First Place 4 Health.

The Bible tells us that Solomon was the wisest man ever to have lived. Read Matthew 12:42 and discuss why Jesus was greater even than Solomon. What were the two types of wisdom that each presented?

On Day One, group members read how God searches us and tests our heart. Talk about the difference between "searching" and "testing."

Talk through the concept of wealth, honor and life. Discuss how each of these terms applies to a person's life in terms of physical and spiritual health.

Read this week's memory verse out loud together. Ask the participants some of the dangers they might encounter as they learn to live a balanced life.

Ask your group to identify some of the things they struggle "keeping on keeping on" with, even though those things may be harmful to their health and fitness goals.

Discuss with participants how children clearly watch and learn from our every move. How might they be influencing their children by the choices they make with regard to food and exercise?

Take some time to identify any faulty messages the members might have received during their formative years. How can they tape over these patterns with God's truth?

When stress is high or emotions set in, it is easy to succumb to that old familiar call to eat more than we need to. Take a look at some of the ways members can remind themselves to lead a peaceful life each day in order to ignore those tempting calls to overeat.

Committing one's plans to the Lord is an important part of healthy living. Spend some time in prayer, asking for guidance in decision-making and peace of mind from worries about the future.

week six: delighting in the Lord

Make sure everyone identified all the "if" and "then" statements in Proverbs 2:1-11, then discuss practical ways they can put these into practice.

Go over the chart used on Day 2 that compares God's attributes with the benefits people reap when living a healthy life.

Summarize what the group has learned about wisdom this summer as it applies to their success in learning to live a balanced life. Be sure to include the benefits of wisdom that will help them reach their physical health and fitness goals as well as the ones that will bring health, healing and balance to them mentally, emotionally and spiritually.

Give each person in your group time to share his or her experiences as he or she has interacted with the material in *Healthy Summer Living*. How has the study of God's Word affected each person's life this summer so far?

Spend some time praying for each other, about the choices they may have made this summer, and about their continued quest to live healthy and balanced lives.

First Place 4 Health summer menus & recipes

Each menu plan is based on approximately 1,400 to 1,500 calories per day. All recipe and menu exchanges were determined using the Master-Cook software, a program that accesses a database containing more than 6,000 food items prepared using the United States Department of Agriculture (USDA) publications and information from food manufacturers. As with any nutritional program, MasterCook calculates the nutritional values of the recipes based on ingredients. Nutrition may vary due to how the food is prepared, where the food comes from, soil content, season, ripeness, processing and method of preparation. For these reasons, please use the recipes and menu plans as approximate guides. Consult a physician and/or a registered dietitian before starting a weight-loss program.

For those who need more calories, add the following to the 1,400-calorie plan:

- 1,800 calories: 2 ounce equivalent of meat, 3 ounce equivalent of bread, $^1/_2$ cup vegetable serving, 1 tsp. fat

- 2,000 calories: 2 ounce equivalent of meat, 4 ounce equivalent of bread, 1/2 cup vegetable serving, 3 tsp. fat

- 2,200 calories: 2 ounce equivalent of meat, 5 ounce equivalent of bread, $^1/_2$ cup vegetable serving, $^1/_2$ cup fruit serving, 5 tsp. fat

- 2,400 calories: 2 ounce equivalent of meat, 6 ounce equivalent of bread, 1 cup vegetable serving, $^1/_2$ cup fruit serving, 6 tsp. fat

First Week Grocery List

Baking Products

- ❏ abodo sauce
- ❏ allspice, ground
- ❏ almonds
- ❏ baking powder
- ❏ baking soda
- ❏ basil, dried and fresh
- ❏ black pepper
- ❏ brown sugar
- ❏ Cajun seasoning
- ❏ caraway seeds
- ❏ cayenne pepper
- ❏ cherry preserves
- ❏ chives, fresh
- ❏ cider vinegar
- ❏ cilantro, fresh
- ❏ cooking oil
- ❏ cumin, ground
- ❏ cumin seeds
- ❏ flour, all-purpose
- ❏ ginger, fresh
- ❏ golden raisins
- ❏ jalapeno chile peppers
- ❏ ketchup
- ❏ lemon juice
- ❏ lime juice, fresh-squeezed
- ❏ marinara sauce
- ❏ mint leaves, fresh
- ❏ olive oil, extra virgin
- ❏ olives
- ❏ oregano, dried
- ❏ parsley
- ❏ peanut butter
- ❏ pimientos
- ❏ plum sauce
- ❏ pumpkin seed kernels, unsalted and toasted
- ❏ raspberry vinegar
- ❏ red pepper, ground
- ❏ red wine vinegar
- ❏ salad dressing, fat-free
- ❏ salsa verde
- ❏ salt
- ❏ semisweet chocolate
- ❏ sugar
- ❏ sugar substitute
- ❏ taco seasoning mix
- ❏ wheat germ, toasted
- ❏ thyme, dried
- ❏ vanilla
- ❏ vegetable oil
- ❏ yeast

Produce

- ❏ (2) apples
- ❏ (2) apricots
- ❏ arugula leaves
- ❏ (2) bananas
- ❏ blueberries
- ❏ coleslaw (1 pkg.)
- ❏ (4) ears corn
- ❏ cucumbers
- ❏ garlic
- ❏ grapes
- ❏ green onions
- ❏ lemon slices
- ❏ mixed greens
- ❏ onions
- ❏ oranges
- ❏ peaches
- ❏ plum tomatoes
- ❏ raspberries
- ❏ red cabbage
- ❏ red onions

❑ red peppers
❑ Savoy cabbage
❑ spinach leaves
❑ strawberries
❑ summer squash, yellow
❑ sweet potatoes
❑ tomatoes
❑ watercress
❑ zucchini

Breads and Cereals
❑ bagel
❑ bread, white (1 pkg.)
❑ bread, whole-wheat (1 pkg.)
❑ hamburger buns, whole grain
  (2 pkgs.)
❑ oats, rolled
❑ pitas (1 pkg.)
❑ pizza dough, whole-wheat
❑ raisin bread
❑ rolls, whole-grain
❑ Shredded Wheat®
❑ spaghetti
❑ tortillas, flour
❑ tortillas, whole-wheat (1 pkg.)

Canned Goods
❑ applesauce, unsweetened (1 jar)
❑ black-eyed peas
❑ chicken broth, reduced-sodium
  (1 can)
❑ chipotle chiles, canned in adobo
  (3 cans)
❑ cream of mushroom soup (1 can)
❑ onions, pickled
❑ refried beans, nonfat (1 can)
❑ turkey, canned (8 ozs.)

Meat and Fish
❑ chicken (small)
❑ (16) chicken breasts, boneless
  and skinless
❑ pork tenderloin (2 lbs.)
❑ roast beef, thinly sliced (8 ozs.)
❑ sirloin, ground (2 lbs.)
❑ turkey, honey-roasted (3 oz.)

Dairy
❑ blue cheese, crumbled (1 ctn.)
❑ butter
❑ cheddar cheese, lowfat (8 ozs.)
❑ cream cheese, light (1 block)
❑ cream cheese, reduced-fat
  (1 block)
❑ eggs
❑ feta cheese, crumbled (1 ctn.)
❑ goat cheese (1 ctn.)
❑ hummus (flavor of your choice)
❑ Laughing Cow® cheese (1 circle)
❑ margarine
❑ milk
❑ part-skim milk mozzarella
  cheese (1 cup)
❑ orange juice
❑ sour cream, light (8-oz. ctn.)
❑ sour cream, nonfat
  (16-oz. ctn.)
❑ yogurt, lowfat vanilla (1 ctn.)
❑ yogurt, lowfat plain (1 ctn.)

Frozen Foods
❑ blueberries, frozen (1 small pkg.)
❑ cherries, frozen (1 small pkg.)
❑ corn, frozen whole-kernel (1 pkg.)
❑ mixed fruit, frozen (2 cups)

First Week Meals and Recipes

DAY 1

....

Breakfast

Vegetable Fritatta with Cheese

8 slightly beaten eggs
1 tbsp. snipped fresh basil or 1 tsp. dried basil, crushed
2 tbsp. olive oil
$^1/_2$ cup chopped zucchini

1 cup frozen whole-kernel corn or cut fresh corn
$^1/_3$ cup thinly sliced green onions
$^3/_4$ cup chopped plum tomatoes
$^1/_2$ cup shredded cheddar cheese

Combine eggs and basil in a medium bowl and set aside. Heat oil in a large skillet; add corn, zucchini and green onions. Cook and stir for 3 minutes, and then add tomatoes. Cook uncovered over medium heat for about 5 minutes or until vegetables are crisp-tender, stirring occasionally. Pour egg mixture over the vegetables in the skillet. Cook over medium heat. As the mixture sets, run a spatula around edge of skillet, lifting egg mixture so that the uncooked portion flows underneath. Continue cooking and lifting edges until this egg mixture is almost set (the surface will be moist). Sprinkle with cheese. Place the skillet under a broiler 4 to 5 inches from heat. Broil 1 to 2 minutes or until the top is just set and the cheese is melted. Serve with 1 cup mixed fruit. Serves 4.

Nutritional Information: 375 calories (51.6% calories from fat); 22g fat; 19g protein; 27g carbohydrate; 3g dietary fiber; 439mg cholesterol; 236mg sodium.

....

Lunch

Asian Chicken Wrap

4 8-inch flour tortillas (preferably whole-wheat)
4 oz. light cream cheese
$^1/_2$ cup Asian plum sauce

3 tbsp. minced peeled fresh ginger
1 small (2-lb.) roasted chicken
1 bunch watercress, stemmed
$^1/_2$ cup chopped green onions

Spread a thin layer of cream cheese on the tortillas and follow with a thin layer of plum sauce. Divide evenly and sprinkle green onions and ginger over tortillas. Cut chicken meat in thin slices and place on top of each tortilla. Lay watercress on top of chicken and roll tortillas into tight rolls. Serves 4.

Note: These are great for a picnic lunch. If you have a fire or outdoor grill at your picnic, grill the tortillas for 2 to 3 minutes until grill marks appear all around them. Remember to store these wraps in your cooler until it is time to serve them.

Nutritional Information: 413 calories (26.4% calories from fat); 12g fat; 21g protein; 54g carbohydrate; 3g dietary fiber; 46mg cholesterol; 670mg sodium.

....

Dinner

Grilled Chicken with Chipotle Barbecue Sauce

1 cup fresh or frozen dark sweet
  cherries, pitted and chopped
$1/_2$ cup reduced-sodium chicken broth
$1/_3$ cup cherry preserves
$1/_3$ cup ketchup
2 tbsp. cider vinegar

$1^1/_2$ tsp. minced canned chipotle
  chiles in adobo sauce
$1^1/_4$ tsp. dried thyme
$1/_2$ tsp. ground allspice
2 lbs. boneless, skinless chicken
  breasts, trimmed of fat

Stir cherries, broth, cherry preserves, ketchup, vinegar, chipotle chiles, thyme and allspice in a small bowl. Transfer to a shallow dish that is large enough to hold the chicken. Add the chicken and turn to coat well. Cover and marinate in the refrigerator for at least 2 hours (or overnight). Preheat the grill to high and oil the grill rack. Remove the chicken from the marinade and transfer the marinade to a medium skillet. Reduce the grill heat to medium and grill the chicken until it is cooked through and no longer pink in the middle (about 7 to 9 minutes per side). Bring the marinade to a boil; reduce heat to a simmer and cook until the sauce is reduced by about half (about 12 to 15 minutes). Let the chicken cool slightly and then serve with the sauce. Serve with 1 cup mixed greens with 2 tablespoons fat-free dressing, one serving of *Oven-Baked Sweet Potato Fries* (see recipe on the next page), and one dinner roll. Serves 8.

Nutritional Information: 180 calories (8.4% calories from fat); 2g fat; 27g protein; 14g carbohydrate; 1g dietary fiber; 66mg cholesterol; 249mg sodium.

Oven-Baked Sweet Potato Fries

$1/2$ tsp. ground cumin	1 tbsp. vegetable oil
$1/2$ tsp. salt	2 large (about $1^1/2$-lb.)
$1/4$ tsp. ground red pepper	sweet potatoes

In a small bowl, combine cumin, salt and red pepper. Set aside. Preheat oven to 400°F. Peel sweet potatoes, cut each in half lengthwise, and then cut each half into 6 wedges. In a large bowl, combine the cut potatoes, oil and spice mixture. Toss until the potatoes are evenly coated. Arrange the potatoes in a single layer on a baking sheet and place the sheet on the middle shelf of the oven. Bake until the edges are crisp and the potatoes are cooked through (about 30 minutes). Serves 4.

Nutritional Information: 99 calories (32.6% calories from fat); 4g fat; 1g protein; 16g carbohydrate; 2g dietary fiber; 0mg cholesterol; 275mg sodium.

DAY 2

Breakfast

Peanut Butter and Banana on Toast

2 tbsp. peanut butter	1 banana
2 slices whole-wheat bread	

Toast the bread and then spread the peanut butter on top. Slice the banana and layer on the peanut butter.

Nutritional Information: 329 calories (48.1% calories from fat); 19g fat; 14g protein; 32g carbohydrate; 6g dietary fiber; 0mg cholesterol; 446mg sodium.

Lunch

Southern Black-eyed Pea Salad

2 tbsp. cooking oil	2 15-oz. cans black-eyed peas,
4 cups yellow summer squash,	rinsed and drained
quartered lengthwise and sliced thin	$1/4$ cup sliced green onions
2 to 4 fresh chopped jalapeno peppers,	2 tbsp. snipped fresh cilantro
seeded, if desired	or parsley

4 cloves garlic, minced
1 tsp. cumin seeds, crushed

$^1/_2$ tsp. salt
2 cups chopped tomatoes

In a large skillet, heat oil over medium heat. Add squash, peppers, garlic and cumin; cook for 5 to 6 minutes or until squash is crisp-tender, stirring occasionally. Remove from heat and cool. In a large bowl, combine squash mixture, black-eyed peas, green onions, cilantro or parsley and salt. Cover and chill. When you are ready to serve, toss the pea mixture together with the 2 cups chopped tomatoes. Serve with whole-wheat crackers or pita bread. Serves 8 ($^3/_4$-cup servings).

Nutritional Information: 205 calories; (18.2% calories from fat); 4g fat; 12g protein; 32g carbohydrate; 7g dietary fiber; 0mg cholesterol; 147mg sodium.

....

Dinner

Grilled Pizza with Garden Tomatoes

1 lb. whole-wheat pizza dough
  or other prepared dough
4 tbsp. prepared tomato sauce
  or marinara sauce
2 lbs. vine-ripened tomatoes,
  thinly sliced (4 to 6 tomatoes)

dash of salt and freshly
  ground pepper, to taste
1 cup grated fresh mozzarella
  cheese
$^1/_4$ cup chopped fresh basil leaves

Prepare the whole-wheat or other prepared dough. If you are cooking the pizzas on a charcoal grill, build a medium-hot fire in one half of the grill (two bricks placed end-to-end work well as a divider). If you are using a gas grill with two burners, preheat one burner on high and leave the other unlit. If you are using a single-burner gas grill, preheat on high and then lower the flame to cook the second side of the pizzas. Roll out the pizza dough into 4 circles and place on a floured cutting board. Put 2 of the dough circles on the hot side of the grill. Within 1 minute, the dough will puff slightly and the underside will firm up and be striped with grill marks. Use tongs to flip the crusts over and onto the cooler side of the grill. Using half of the ingredients, spread tomato sauce or marinara sauce on the crusts after you turn them and then cover with overlapping tomato slices. Sprinkle salt and pepper and scatter mozzarella over all. Cover the grill and cook, rotating the pizzas once or twice until the toppings are heated through (about 5 minutes). Remove the pizzas from the grill. Repeat with the remaining dough and toppings. Just before serving, sprinkle the pizzas with basil. Serve with 2 cups fresh spinach, sliced tomatoes, cucumber and fat-free dressing. Serves: 4 (one 6-inch pizza each).

Nutritional Information: 385 calories (40% of calories from fat); 17g fat (4g saturated fat and 3g monounsaturated fat); 16g protein; 44g carbohydrate; 7g fiber; 18mg cholesterol; 785mg sodium.

DAY 3

Breakfast

McDonald's Egg McMuffin®   1 cup milk
1 small apple

Nutritional Information: 467 calories (24.5% calories from fat); 13g fat; 27g protein; 63g carbohydrate; 6g dietary fiber; 264mg cholesterol; 946mg sodium.

Lunch

Honey-Roasted Turkey Wrap with Hummus
1 whole-wheat tortilla $^1/_4$ cup hummus
3 oz. honey-roasted turkey   4 to 6 large spinach leaves,
  (thin sliced)   with stems removed

Cover tortilla with a layer of hummus. Cover evenly with sliced turkey and place the spinach leaves lengthwise down the center. Roll the tortilla tightly, wrap in plastic and chill until set (about 30 minutes). Cut the roll into $1^1/_2$-inch thick slices. Store in a resealable container and keep cool until you are ready to serve. Serve with one fresh peach. Serves 13.

Nutritional Information: 347 calories; (28.7% calories from fat); 11g fat; 12g protein; 50g carbohydrate; 7g dietary fiber; 0mg cholesterol; 613mg sodium.

Dinner

Chipotle-Marinated Pork Tenderloin
2 canned chipotle chiles   1 tsp. dried oregano
1 tsp. adobo sauce $^1/_2$ tsp. ground cumin
1 clove of garlic, minced $^1/_4$ tsp. salt

¹/₂ cup orange juice
3 tbsp. lime juice
1 tbsp. red wine vinegar

¹/₄ tsp. freshly ground pepper
2 lbs. pork tenderloin,
  trimmed of fat

Combine chipotle and adobo sauce, garlic, orange juice, lime juice, vinegar, oregano, cumin, salt and pepper in a blender. Blend until the chipotle is chopped and the mixture is relatively smooth. Pour the mixture into a sealable plastic bag, add pork and then seal, squeezing out any excess air from the bag. Turn to coat with the marinade. Refrigerate at least 1 hour and up to 8 hours. Preheat grill to high or heat a large indoor grill pan over high heat. Remove the pork from the marinade (discard the marinade). Grill the pork, turning occasionally, until the meat reaches a temperature of 145°F (about 12 to 15 minutes). Transfer the pork to a cutting board and let it sit for 5 minutes before slicing. Serve with 1 cup cooked carrots, 1 dinner roll and 2 cups of mixed greens with fat-free dressing. Serves 4. (*Note:* reserve half of the cooked pork for lunch next week, or freeze for up to three months.)

Nutritional Information: 158 calories (23.3% calories from fat); 4g fat; 25g protein; 5g carbohydrate; 1g dietary fiber; 74mg cholesterol; 236mg sodium.

DAY 4

Breakfast

Spinach Omelet
nonstick cooking spray
4 eggs or 1 cup refrigerated or
  frozen egg product, thawed
dash of salt
dash of cayenne pepper
1 cup spinach leaves

¹/₄ cup shredded sharp
  cheddar cheese
1 tbsp. snipped fresh chives,
  flat-leaf parsley or chervil
Red Pepper Relish (recipe on the
  following page)

Lightly coat an 8-inch nonstick skillet with flared sides or a crepe pan with nonstick cooking spray. Heat skillet over medium-high heat. In a medium bowl, beat together eggs, salt and cayenne pepper with a rotary beater or wire whisk until frothy. Pour into the prepared skillet and cook over medium heat. As egg mixture sets, run a spatula around edge of skillet, lifting the egg mixture so that the uncooked portion flows underneath. Continue cooking and lifting edges until the egg mixture is set but still glossy and moist. Sprinkle with cheese and chives, parsely or chervil. Top with $^3/_4$ cup of the spinach leaves and 2 tablespoons of the *Red Pepper Relish*. Lift and fold an edge of the omelet partially over filling. Top with the remaining $^1/_4$ cup spinach and 1 tablespoon of the relish (you can keep the remaining relish for another use). Cut the omelet in half and serve with 1 cup sliced melon. Serves 2.

Nutritional Information: 456 calories (58.7% calories from fat); 30g fat; 34g protein; 13g carbohydrate; 3g dietary fiber; 878mg cholesterol; 749mg sodium.

Red Pepper Relish

$^2/_3$ cup red sweet pepper, chopped
2 tbsp. finely chopped onion

1 tbsp. cider vinegar
$^1/_4$ tsp. black pepper

Combine red sweet pepper, onion, vinegar and black pepper in a small bowl. Makes about $^2/_3$ cup.

....

Lunch

Grilled Chicken Salad with Goat Cheese and Raspberry Vinaigrette

nonstick cooking spray
4 boneless, skinless chicken breasts
 (about 4 oz. each)
dash of salt
dash of freshly ground black pepper
$^1/_4$ cup raspberry vinegar

$^1/_2$ tsp. sugar
2 tbsp. extra virgin olive oil
8 cups mixed baby greens
$^1/_2$ cup golden raisins
4 tbsp. goat cheese
1 cup raspberries

Spray a grill grate or broiler pan with nonstick spray and preheat the grill or broiler to medium-high. Season the chicken breasts with salt and pepper. Grill or broil the chicken until it is cooked through (about 6 minutes per side). Remove the chicken from the grill and let cool. (*Note:* You can do this in advance and store the chicken in a refrigerator for up to 3 days.) Slice the chicken into strips. Whisk the vinegar, sugar and olive oil together in a large salad bowl and season with salt and pepper. Add the greens and toss to coat the greens with dressing. Arrange the sliced chicken and place the raisins, goat cheese and raspberries on top. Serves 4.

Nutritional Information: 462 calories (24.5% calories from fat); 13g fat; 61g protein; 27g carbohydrate; 7g dietary fiber; 144mg cholesterol; 209mg sodium.

DAY 5

Breakfast

$^1/_2$ cup Shredded Wheat® with
  1 cup lowfat milk
1 slice raisin toast with
  1 tbsp. cream cheese

1 sliced peach

Nutritional Information: 263 calories (14.0% calories from fat); 4g fat; 13g protein; 45g carbohydrate; 5g dietary fiber; 12mg cholesterol; 307mg sodium.

Lunch

Cool Cucumber Cheese Sandwich

1 large cucumber
4 oz. reduced-fat cream cheese
  (Neufchatel)
2 tbsp. fresh basil
8 slices firm-textured whole-
  wheat bread
$^1/_8$ tsp. salt, if desired

2 large apricots or 1 nectarine,
  pitted and thinly sliced
$^1/_2$ cup arugula leaves or
  cilantro sprigs

Peel cucumber, cut in half lengthwise and scoop out the seeds. Thinly slice the cucumber and set aside. In a small bowl, stir together the cream cheese, basil and, if desired, salt. Spread about 1 tablespoon of the cream cheese mixture on one side of each slice of bread. Top four of the bread slices with cucumber, apricot and arugula leaves or cilantro sprigs. Top with the remaining bread slices, cream cheese side down, to make 4 sandwiches. Cut each sandwich in half diagonally. Serve with 1 cup grapes. Serves 4.

Nutritional Information: 222 calories (29.1% calories from fat); 8g fat; 9g protein; 32g carbohydrate; 5g dietary fiber; 16mg cholesterol; 457mg sodium.

Dinner

Turkey Spaghetti

nonstick cooking spray
$^1/_2$ cup chopped onion
8 ozs. diced turkey
1 can cream of mushroom soup,
  lowfat
2 cups spaghetti, cooked

4 oz. reduced-fat cheddar cheese,
  shredded
1 small jar pimientos, chopped
1 tsp. dried parsley flakes
dash of pepper

Spray large skillet with nonstick cooking spray. Sauté onion with turkey and blend in mushroom soup and cheddar cheese. Cook over low heat until the cheese is melted, stirring constantly. Add cooked spaghetti, pimientos, parsley flakes and pepper and pour in a baking dish. Bake at 350°F for 14 minutes. Serve with mixed green salad and dinner roll. Serves 4.

Nutritional Information: 340 calories (23.9% calories from fat); 9g fat; 27g protein; 37g carbohydrate; 2g dietary fiber; 44mg cholesterol; 701mg sodium.

DAY 6

Breakfast

Blueberry Oat Muffins

$1^1/_2$ cups all-purpose flour
$^3/_4$ cup rolled oats
2 tsp. baking powder
$^1/_2$ tsp. baking soda
$^1/_4$ tsp. salt
1 egg, beaten

$^3/_4$ cup milk
$^1/_2$ cup packed brown sugar
$^1/_4$ cup cooking oil
$^1/_2$ tsp. vanilla
$^3/_4$ cup fresh or frozen blueberries

Grease 12 $2^1/_2$-inch muffin cups and set aside. Stir together flour, rolled oats, baking powder, baking soda and salt in a bowl. Make a well in the center of the mixture. Combine egg, milk, brown sugar, oil and vanilla in another bowl. Add egg mixture all at once to the flour mixture. Stir until moistened (the batter should be lumpy) and then fold in blueberries. Spoon the batter into the prepared muffin cups, filling each three-quarters full. Bake at 400°F for 16 to 18 minutes. Cool muffin cups on a wire rack for 5 minutes and then remove from the cups. Serve warm. Serve with a banana and 1 cup lowfat milk. Makes 12 muffins.

Nutritional Information: 172 calories (31.1% calories from fat); 6g fat; 3g protein; 26g carbohydrate; 1g dietary fiber; 20mg cholesterol; 196mg sodium.

....

Lunch

1 Arby's Regular Roast
   Beef Sandwich®
1 orange

Tossed salad with
   2-3 tbsp. fat-free salad dressing

Nutritional Information: 431 calories (36.6% calories from fat); 18g fat; 22g protein; 48g carbohydrate; 3g dietary fiber; 37mg cholesterol; 1,321mg sodium.

....

Dinner

Backyard Coleslaw
2 tbsp. extra virgin olive oil
2 tbsp. red wine vinegar
1 tsp. sugar
$1/2$ tsp. caraway seeds, crushed
dash of salt
dash of freshly ground pepper

3 cups finely shredded
   Savoy cabbage
3 cups finely shredded red
   cabbage, rinsed
$1/3$ cup coarsely grated onion

Whisk oil, vinegar, sugar, caraway seeds, salt and pepper in a large bowl. Add Savoy cabbage, red cabbage and onion. Toss to coat. Serve within 2 hours. Serves 4.

Nutritional Information: 66 calories (90.1% calories from fat); 7g fat; trace protein; 2g carbohydrate; trace dietary fiber; 0mg cholesterol; 33mg sodium.

Grilled Corn on the Cob
4 ears of corn, unhusked

Preheat grill. Carefully peel back husks, but do not detach. Remove as much silk from the ears of corn as possible. Pull the husks back over the corn and secure the end by tying with a strip of husk. Soak the corn in cold water for 20 minutes. Remove from the water, shaking off excess. Grill the ears of corn, periodically rolling them for even cooking, until the kernels are tender when pierced with a fork (about 15 to 20 minutes). Remove the husks before serving.

Nutritional Information: 77 calories (10.7% calories from fat); 1g fat; 3g protein; 17g carbohydrate; 2g dietary fiber; 0mg cholesterol; 14mg sodium.

Blue-Cheese Burgers

nonstick cooking spray	$1/2$ tsp. black pepper
2 1-oz. slices of country white bread	2 lbs. lean ground sirloin
2 tbsp. fat-free milk	$1/2$ cup crumbled blue cheese
$1/2$ tsp. salt	8 hamburger rolls, halved

Prepare the grill by spraying the rack with nonstick cooking spray. Place bread in a blender and blend for 30 seconds or until finely ground. Place breadcrumbs in a large bowl and add milk; toss with a fork to moisten. Add salt, pepper and ground sirloin to the breadcrumb mixture, stirring just until combined. Divide the meat mixture into 16 equal portions, shaping each into a $3^{1}/_{2}$-inch patty. Spoon 1 tablespoon blue cheese in the center of each of the 8 patties and top each with a remaining patty, pinching edges to seal. Place patties on the grill rack coated with cooking spray; grill 4 minutes on each side. Remove from heat and keep warm. Lightly coat cut sides of rolls with cooking spray; place cut sides down on grill rack and grill for 30 seconds or until toasted. Serve patties on toasted rolls with desired toppings. Serves 8.

Nutritional Information: 437 calories (50.9% calories from fat); 24g fat; 27g protein; 25g carbohydrate; 1g dietary fiber; 85mg cholesterol; 602mg sodium.

DAY 7

Breakfast

$1/2$ large bagel	1 cup mixed fruit
1 tbsp. reduced-fat cream cheese	

Nutritional Information: 400 calories (8.0% calories from fat); 4g fat; 10g protein; 85g carbohydrate; 6g dietary fiber; 8mg cholesterol; 325mg sodium.

....

Lunch

Roast Beef Sandwiches with Sweet and Sour Red Onions and Blue Cheese

2 cups thinly sliced red onions	$1/2$ cup crumbled blue cheese
2 tbsp. red wine vinegar	12 tomato slices
1 tsp. sugar	8 oz. thinly sliced roast beef
dash of salt and pepper	2 cups (packed) small watercress
4 large soft whole-grain rolls,	sprigs
toasted	1 cup pickled onions

Combine onions, vinegar and sugar in medium bowl and sprinkle with salt and pepper. Let stand until the onions are soft, tossing occasionally, at least 1 hour and up to 4 hours. Place bottom halves of the whole grain rolls on work surface and sprinkle with cheese. Top each half with 3 tomato slices and $1/4$ of the roast beef. Top each with $1/2$ cup watercress and $1/4$ cup pickled onions. Cover with tops of rolls. Cut each sandwich in half and serve with one fresh peach. Serves 4.

Nutritional Information: 341 calories (41.2% calories from fat); 16g fat; 19g protein; 33g carbohydrate; 6g dietary fiber; 45mg cholesterol; 540mg sodium.

....

Dinner

Grilled Chicken Tostadas

4 6-oz. skinless, boneless	1 7-oz. can green salsa
chicken breast halves	4 cups chopped tomato
1 tbsp. fresh lime juice	$1/4$ cup sliced ripe olives, chopped
1 tbsp. 40-percent less-sodium	$1 1/4$ cups fat-free refried beans
taco seasoning	$1/2$ cup crumbled feta cheese
$1/2$ tsp. sugar	6 tbsp. reduced-fat sour cream
nonstick cooking spray	$1/4$ cup fresh cilantro leaves
6 8-inch flour tortillas	$1/4$ cup unsalted pumpkin
6 cups packaged coleslaw	seed kernels, toasted

Prepare grill or heat a grill pan over medium-high heat. Brush chicken with lime juice and sprinkle with taco seasoning and sugar. Place the chicken on grill rack or in a grill pan coated with nonstick cooking spray and grill 4 minutes on each side until chicken is done. Cool slightly. Cut chicken into

$1/_4$-inch strips and set aside. Place tortillas on the grill rack or pan and grill 30 seconds on each side or until golden brown. In a small bowl, combine coleslaw and salsa and toss to coat. Combine tomato and olives in a separate bowl and toss gently. Spread about 3 tablespoons of the refried beans over each tortilla and divide chicken evenly among the tortillas. Top each serving with $2/_3$ cup of the slaw mixture, $2/_3$ cup of the tomato mixture, 4 teaspoons feta cheese, 1 tablespoon reduced-fat sour cream and 2 teaspoons cilantro leaves. Sprinkle each serving with 2 teaspoons pumpkin seeds, if desired.

Nutritional Information: 361 calories (22.9% of calories from fat); 9.2g fat; 28.7g protein; 43g carbohydrate; 6.8g dietary fiber; 65g cholesterol; 844mg sodium.

Second Week Grocery List

Produce
- ☐ (2) apples
- ☐ asparagus, fresh
- ☐ (2) bananas
- ☐ basil, fresh ($^1/_3$ cup)
- ☐ black raspberries ($^1/_4$ cup)
- ☐ carrots, baby (1 bag)
- ☐ cherry tomatoes (1 pkg.)
- ☐ (2) cucumbers
- ☐ (2) eggplants
- ☐ garlic (2 cloves)
- ☐ (2) green bell peppers
- ☐ (2) honeydew melon
- ☐ lemon juice
- ☐ (2) lemons
- ☐ mixed salad greens (2 bags)
- ☐ (2) onions
- ☐ peach
- ☐ (3) plum tomatoes
- ☐ (3) red onions
- ☐ (2) red peppers
- ☐ strawberries ($^1/_2$ cup)
- ☐ thyme leaf, fresh
- ☐ (5) tomatoes
- ☐ watermelon
- ☐ yellow onions
- ☐ yellow squash
- ☐ (2) zucchini

Breads and Cereals
- ☐ (2) bagels
- ☐ baked chips
- ☐ bread crumbs
- ☐ buns, whole-wheat (1 pkg.)
- ☐ cornflakes
- ☐ English muffins
- ☐ French bread (1 loaf)
- ☐ graham crackers
- ☐ oats, steel-cut
- ☐ pita bread rounds (1 pkg.)
- ☐ wheat germ, toasted

Baking Products
- ☐ almonds ($^1/_3$ cup)
- ☐ balsamic vinegar
- ☐ barbecue sauce
- ☐ black olives, sliced (1 small can)
- ☐ brown rice
- ☐ canola oil
- ☐ cayenne
- ☐ cider vinegar
- ☐ cinnamon, ground
- ☐ cola, diet (with saccharin)
- ☐ cranberries, dried
- ☐ cumin, ground
- ☐ dijon mustard
- ☐ dried fruit
- ☐ garlic powder
- ☐ honey
- ☐ Italian dressing, fat-free
- ☐ maple syrup, sugar-free
- ☐ marmalade, orange
- ☐ mayonnaise, lowfat
- ☐ mint, fresh
- ☐ mustard
- ☐ olive oil
- ☐ oregano, dried
- ☐ paprika
- ☐ peanut butter
- ☐ pecans ($^1/_4$ cup)

- [ ] pepper (ground)
- [ ] poppy seeds
- [ ] pumpkin pie spice
- [ ] ranch dressing, fat-free
- [ ] red wine vinegar
- [ ] salad dressing, fat-free
- [ ] salad dressing, reduced-calorie
- [ ] salsa
- [ ] salt
- [ ] sugar
- [ ] thyme, dried
- [ ] tomatoes, sun-dried
- [ ] vinegar, fruit-flavored
- [ ] walnuts ($^1/_2$ cup)
- [ ] wooden skewers
- [ ] Worcestershire sauce

Dairy

- [ ] eggs
- [ ] feta cheese, crumbled (1 pkg.)
- [ ] margarine, light
- [ ] milk, lowfat
- [ ] milk, nonfat
- [ ] orange juice
- [ ] sour cream, light
- [ ] yogurt, lowfat vanilla (1 ctn.)

- [ ] yogurt, plain lowfat (1 ctn.)
- [ ] yogurt, nonfat sugar-free vanilla (1 ctn.)

Canned Foods

- [ ] applesauce, unsweetened (1 small jar)
- [ ] chipotle chiles canned in adobo (2 cans)
- [ ] mandarin oranges, in water (4-oz. can)
- [ ] mixed fruit (15-oz. can)
- [ ] tomato soup (2 cans)

Seafood and Meat

- [ ] beef sirloin (1 lb.)
- [ ] (4) catfish fillets
- [ ] (2) chicken breast halves (2 cups)
- [ ] (4) chicken breasts, boneless and skinless
- [ ] (4) cod fillets, frozen
- [ ] ground round (1 lb.)
- [ ] pork tenderloin (2 lbs.)

Frozen Foods

- [ ] Stouffer's Lean Cuisine Cheese Cannelloni®
- [ ] waffles, whole-wheat frozen

Second Week Meals and Recipes

DAY 1

Breakfast

1 serving cornflakes or other
  low-sugar cereal

1 cup milk
1 sliced banana

Nutritional Information: 347 calories (3.2% calories from fat); 1g fat; 12g protein; 76g carbohydrate; 4g dietary fiber; 4mg cholesterol; 574mg sodium.

Lunch

Chipotle Pork Sandwich

1 tsp. canola oil
1 small yellow onion,
  cut into $^1/_2$-inch-thick rounds
4 whole-wheat buns, split horizontally

1 lb. uncooked pork (or use $^1/_2$
  of the *Chipotle-Marinated Pork
  Tenderloin* from last week)
$^1/_3$ cup barbecue sauce

Preheat grill to high or heat a large indoor grill pan over high heat. Lightly brush onion with canola oil and grill until lightly browned and soft, turning once (about 4 to 5 minutes). Let cool on a cutting board. Lightly toast buns cut side down on the grill or in the pan. Chop the onion and transfer to a large saucepan. Shred the pork tenderloins using two forks and add to the onions. Add barbecue sauce and stir to combine. Heat over low heat until warm throughout. Put the pork filling on the toasted buns. Serve with 1 cup baby carrots with fat-free ranch dressing. Serves 4.

Nutritional Information: 334 calories (20.9% calories from fat); 8g fat; 30g protein; 34g carbohydrate; 4g dietary fiber; 74mg cholesterol; 577mg sodium.

Dinner

2 slices Thin-n-Crispy Pizza Hut
  Pizza Supreme® ($^1/_3$ of a
  10″ pizza)

1 tossed salad
1 tbsp. fat-free salad dressing
$^1/_2$ cup fresh mixed fruit

Nutritional Information: 572 calories (18.1% calories from fat); 12g fat; 27g protein; 100g carbohydrate; 10g dietary fiber; 40mg cholesterol; 16,72mg sodium.

DAY 2

....

Breakfast

Swiss Oatmeal

$1^1/_2$ cups water
$^3/_4$ cup steel-cut oats
$^3/_4$ cup fat-free milk
1 6-oz. carton plain lowfat yogurt
3 tbsp. honey
$^1/_4$ tsp. apple pie or pumpkin
  pie spice
$^1/_3$ cup coarsely chopped
  almonds, toasted

$^1/_2$ cup assorted dried fruit
  (such as cranberries, blueberries,
  apples, apricots or plums and/or
  dried fruit bits)
$^1/_8$ tsp. salt

Combine water and oats in a 2-quart saucepan. Bring to boiling and reduce heat. Simmer, uncovered, for 8 minutes (oats will not be tender). Remove from heat and transfer to a mixing bowl. Cool for 5 minutes and then stir in milk, yogurt, 2 tablespoons of the honey, apple pie or pumpkin spice, salt and dried fruits. Cover and chill 12 hours (up to 3 days). When ready to serve, heat oatmeal in saucepan over low heat for 10 minutes. Stir in the remaining 1 tablespoon honey and divide among the serving bowls. Top with almonds and sliced banana. Serve $^2/_3$ cup of the oatmeal with 1 cup blueberries and 1 cup lowfat milk. Makes $3^1/_4$ cups.

Nutritional Information: 211 calories (27.3% calories from fat); 7g fat; 8g protein; 32g carbohydrate; 3g dietary fiber; 4mg cholesterol; 113mg sodium.

....

Lunch

1 Stouffer's Lean Cuisine
  Frozen Dinner Entrée®
1 small apple

1 cup fresh baby carrots with
  2 oz. fat-free ranch dressing

Nutritional Information: 401 calories (20.4% calories from fat); 9g fat; 11g protein; 65g carbohydrate; 11g dietary fiber; 20mg cholesterol; 773mg sodium.

(*Note:* This information is based on Lean Cuisine Cheese Cannelloni® and may vary according to the entrée chosen.)

Dinner

Beef and Vegetable Kebabs

1¹/₂ cups cooked brown rice
2 cups water
4 oz. top sirloin
3 tbsp. fat-free Italian dressing
nonstick cooking spray
4 cherry tomatoes

1 green bell pepper, seeded and
 cut into 4 pieces
1 small onion, cut into 4 wedges
2 wooden skewers, soaked in water
 for 30 minutes, or metal skewers

In a saucepan, combine the rice and water over high heat. Bring to a boil. Reduce the heat to low and then cover and simmer until the water is absorbed and the rice is tender (about 30 to 45 minutes). Add more water if necessary to keep the rice from drying out. Transfer to a small bowl to keep the rice warm. Cut the sirloin into 4 equal portions. Put the meat into a small bowl and pour the Italian dressing over the top. Place in the refrigerator for at least 20 minutes to marinate, turning as needed. Prepare a hot fire in a charcoal grill or heat a gas grill or a broiler. Lightly coat the grill rack or broiler pan away from the heat source with cooking spray. Position the cooking rack 4 to 6 inches from the heat source. Thread 2 cubes of the meat, 2 green pepper slices, 2 cherry tomatoes and 2 onion wedges onto each skewer. Place the kebabs on the grill rack or broiler pan. Grill or broil the kebabs for about 5 to 10 minutes, turning as needed. Divide the rice onto individual plates and top with 1 kebab. Serve with dinner roll and 1 cup steamed asparagus. Serves 2.

Nutritional Information: 333 calories (26.1% calories from fat); 10g fat; 15g protein; 46g carbohydrate; 3g dietary fiber; 36mg cholesterol; 43mg sodium.

DAY 3

Breakfast

Cool and Fruity Breakfast Parfait

1 1¹/₂" graham cracker
 square, crumbled
8 oz. nonfat, sugar-free
 vanilla yogurt
4 walnut halves, chopped

¹/₂ cup strawberries, sliced or
¹/₂ cup blueberries
3 tbsp. wheat germ or 2 tbsp.
 Double Oat Granola (see
 snack recipes)

Alternate ingredients by layering in parfait dish.

Nutritional Information: 382 calories (38.1% calories from fat); 17g fat; 19g protein; 43g carbohydrate; 6g dietary fiber; 3mg cholesterol; 175mg sodium.

....

Lunch

Picnic Pitas

3 tbsp. balsamic or red wine vinegar
2 tsp. olive oil
$1/_4$ cup fresh, chopped basil
1 small eggplant, sliced into
    thin rounds
1 zucchini, sliced thinly
1 yellow squash, sliced thinly
1 red pepper, sliced thinly

1 small red onion, sliced thinly
$1/_4$ cup lowfat plain yogurt
2 tbsp. lowfat mayonnaise
1 tbsp. fresh, chopped basil
1 tsp. lemon juice
4 pitas halves, crusty rolls or
    Focaccia bread

Preheat oven to 450°F. Blend vinegar, oil and basil. Add eggplant, zucchini, squash, red pepper and red onion, tossing to coat. Place vegetables in roasting pan and cook, stirring occasionally until tender (about 30 minutes). In a small bowl, whisk together yogurt, mayonnaise, basil and lemon juice. Spread yogurt mixture on pita halves, crusty rolls or Focaccia bread. Top with veggie mixture and serve with 1 cup of watermelon cubes and *Peachy Lemonade* (see snack recipes).

Nutritional Information: 283 calories; (18.5% calories from fat); 6g fat; 9g protein; 51g carbohydrate; 7g dietary fiber; 4mg cholesterol; 372mg sodium.

....

Dinner

Baked Cod

3 oz. frozen cod
2 tbsp. yogurt
1 tsp. mustard spread
$1/_2$ cup cooked asparagus
1 lemon wedge

$2/_3$ cup cooked rice
1 tossed salad
2 tbsp. reduced-calorie dressing
$1/_4$ cup water-packed mandarin
    orange sections, drained

Spread the yogurt and mustard spread on the cod before baking. Bake the cod per the package instructions. Cook the asparagus and rice in separate saucepans; combine and add lemon wedge. Serve with tossed salad, dressing and mandarin orange sections. Serves 1.

Nutritional Information: 333 calories (7.7% calories from fat); 2g fat; 11g protein; 56g carbohydrate; 6g dietary fiber; 4mg cholesterol; 229mg sodium.

DAY 4

Breakfast

$^1/_2$ English muffin, toasted, with   1 cup nonfat milk
  1 tbsp. peanut butter and $^1/_2$ banana

Nutritional Information: 302 calories (27.1% calories from fat); 9g fat; 15g protein; 42g carbohydrate; 3g dietary fiber; 4mg cholesterol; 334mg sodium.

Lunch

Chicken and Fruit Salad

2 cups boneless, skinless $^1/_4$ tsp. salt
  chicken breasts   dash of freshly ground pepper
$^1/_4$ cup chopped walnuts, toasted   8 cups mixed salad greens
$^1/_4$ cup reduced-fat sour cream   2 cups chopped melon (such as
3 tbsp. fruit-flavored vinegar   cantaloupe or honeydew)
4 tsp. sugar $^1/_4$ cup crumbled feta cheese
$1^1/_2$ tsp. poppy seeds

Place chicken breasts in a medium skillet or saucepan and add lightly salted water. Bring to a boil. Cover, reduce heat to low and simmer gently until chicken is cooked through and no longer pink in the middle (about 10 to 12 minutes). Heat a small dry skillet over medium-low heat. Add walnuts and cook, stirring constantly, until lightly browned and fragrant (about 2 to 3 minutes). Whisk sour cream, vinegar, sugar, poppy seeds, salt and pepper together in a large bowl until smooth. Place $^1/_4$ cup of the dressing in a small bowl. Add the mixed salad greens to the large bowl and toss to coat. Divide among 4 plates and top with chicken, melon, walnuts and feta cheese. Drizzle each portion with 1 tablespoon of the dressing placed at the side. Serve with crackers or *Blueberry Oat Muffin* (see recipe from last week).

Nutritional Information: 339 calories (39.0% calories from fat); 15g fat; 34g protein; 18g carbohydrate; 3g dietary fiber; 90mg cholesterol; 347mg sodium.

Dinner

2 Taco Bell Spicy Chicken
  Soft Tacos®

3 tbsp. salsa
1 medium peach or apple

Nutritional Information: 396 calories (25.7% calories from fat); 12g fat; 21g protein; 58g carbohydrate; 7g dietary fiber; 50mg cholesterol; 1,509mg sodium.

DAY 5

Breakfast

2 whole-wheat frozen waffles
1 tsp. light margarine
2 tsp. sugar-free maple syrup

1 cup honeydew melon
1 cup nonfat milk

Nutritional Information: 337 calories (20.9% calories from fat); 8g fat; 13g protein; 54g carbohydrate; 3g dietary fiber; 27mg cholesterol; 713mg sodium.

Lunch

Quick and Light Greek Salad

2 cucumbers
3/4 cup crumbled, reduced-fat feta
  cheese (or substitute blue cheese)
1/2 cup sliced, canned black
  olives, drained
2/3 cup chopped red onion

3 cups diced Roma tomatoes
  (or another type of vine-ripened
  tomato, or cherry tomato halves)
1/3 cup julienne sun-dried
  tomatoes, oil lightly drained off

Slice the cucumbers into halves, remove the seeds (also remove the peel if desired), and then slice into wedges. In a salad bowl, combine cucumbers, feta cheese, olives, tomatoes and onion, and gently toss. Cover bowl and chill in refrigerator. Serve with slice of warm French bread. Serves 8.

Nutritional Information: 354 calories (23.3% calories from fat); 10g fat; 13g protein; 64g carbohydrate; 17g dietary fiber; trace cholesterol; 1,008mg sodium.

Dinner

Sloppy Joes

1 lb. ground round, select grade
1 large green bell pepper, chopped

1 large onion, chopped
6 whole-wheat hamburger buns

1¹/₂ cans (10³/₄-oz. each) reduced-sodium tomato soup

1 cup mixed melon cubes

1 oz. baked chips

Cook the ground beef, pepper and onion in a nonstick frying pan until the meat is browned and the vegetables are tender (about 7 to 10 minutes). Drain and return the mixture to the frying pan. Add the tomato soup to the ground beef mixture and stir well; simmer for at least 10 minutes. When ready to serve, place ²/₃ cup of the mixture on each hamburger bun. Serve with melon cubes and baked chips. Serves 6.

Nutritional Information: 324 calories (44.3% calories from fat); 16g fat; 19g protein; 26g carbohydrate; 2g dietary fiber; 52mg cholesterol; 422mg sodium.

DAY 6

Breakfast

Berry Banana Smoothie
1 small banana, peeled, cut and frozen
¹/₄ cup fresh or frozen assorted berries (such as raspberries, blackberries or strawberries)

1 cup orange juice
3 tbsp. vanilla lowfat yogurt
fresh mint (optional)

Combine the frozen banana pieces, fresh or frozen berries, orange juice and yogurt in a blender. Cover and blend until smooth. If desired, garnish smoothies with fresh mint and additional berries. Makes 2 (8-oz.) servings.

Nutritional Information: 272 calories (5.4% calories from fat); 2g fat; 5g protein; 63g carbohydrate; 5g dietary fiber; 2mg cholesterol; 32mg sodium.

Lunch

McDonald's® hamburger with small fries
diet soda

tossed green salad with fat-free salad dressing

Nutritional Information: 481 calories (39% of calories from fat); 20.5g fat, 14.8g protein; 60g carbohydrate; 4.8g dietary fiber; 25mg cholesterol; 681mg sodium.

Dinner

Chicken Breasts Glazed with Sweet Marmalade

2 tbsp. olive oil
1 egg
4 boneless and skinless chicken
  breast halves, pounded to
  $1/_4$-inch thickness
$1/_2$ cup bread crumbs

$1/_4$ cup orange marmalade
1 tsp. fresh lemon juice
$1/_4$ tsp. Worcestershire sauce
$1/_4$ tsp. dijon mustard

Heat the olive oil in a medium skillet over medium-high heat. Beat the egg in a shallow bowl; dip chicken breast halves in egg, and then in bread crumbs to coat. Cook the chicken in the skillet for 2 to 4 minutes per side. To create the glaze, combine marmalade, lemon juice, Worcestershire sauce, dijon mustard and garlic together in a bowl and then spread over the chicken. Reduce heat to low and continue cooking the chicken for 4 to 5 minutes, or until glaze color is dulled. Serve with mixed greens with fat-free dressing and $1/_2$ cup rice pilaf. Serves 4.

Nutritional Information: 391 calories (27.9% calories from fat); 12g fat; 58g protein; 10g carbohydrate; trace dietary fiber; 190mg cholesterol; 287mg sodium.

DAY 7

Breakfast

1 small 2-oz. bagel, toasted and
  topped with 1 tsp. light margarine

1 cup mixed fruit

Nutritional Information: 384 calories (6.8% calories from fat); 3g fat; 8g protein; 84g carbohydrate; 6g dietary fiber; 0mg cholesterol; 291mg sodium.

Lunch

Roasted Vegetable Sub

nonstick cooking spray
1 small eggplant, cut in 1-inch pieces
1 small zucchini or yellow summer
  squash, cut into $3/_4$-inch slices
1 tbsp. olive oil

$1/_8$ tsp. salt
2 medium plum tomatoes,
  each cut lengthwise into 6 wedges
1 clove garlic, halved
$1/_2$ tsp. dried thyme, crushed

1 medium red sweet pepper,
  cut in strips
1/2 of a small red onion,
  cut in 1/2-inch wedges
fresh thyme sprigs (optional)

8 small or 4 large 1/2-inch slices
  whole-wheat or white French bread
  (about 8 oz. total), toasted
2 tbsp. balsamic vinegar

Preheat oven to 400°F. Coat a large shallow roasting pan with nonstick cooking spray and add eggplant, zucchini, sweet pepper and onion. Drizzle in olive oil and sprinkle in crushed thyme, salt and pepper. Toss to coat. Roast vegetables for 30 minutes, tossing once. Add tomatoes to roasting pan and roast 15 to 20 minutes more, or until vegetables are tender and some surface areas are lightly browned. Rub toasted bread with cut sides of the garlic clove. Place two small slices or one large slice of the bread on four serving plates. Sprinkle balsamic vinegar over vegetables and toss gently to coat. Spoon warm vegetables on bread and, if desired, garnish with fresh thyme sprigs. Serve with one cup of mixed fruit. Serves 4.

Nutritional Information: 402 calories (16.0% calories from fat); 7g fat; 13g protein; 73g carbohydrate; 8g dietary fiber; 0mg cholesterol; 700mg sodium.

....

Dinner

Blackened Catfish
2 tsp. paprika
1 tsp. garlic powder
1 tsp. dried thyme
1 tsp. salt

1 tsp. finely grated lemon zest
1 tbsp. olive oil
4 catfish fillets (about 4 oz. each)
2 tbsp. lemon juice

In a large shallow dish, combine the paprika, cayenne, garlic powder, thyme, salt and lemon zest. Add the catfish fillets and turn to coat both sides, pressing the herb-and-spice rub into the fish. Heat the olive oil in a large nonstick frying pan over medium-high heat. Add the fish and cook for four minutes. Pour the lemon juice over the fillets, and then turn and cook until the fish just separates when pressed with a fork (about 4 minutes more). Serve with 1/2 cup garlic mashed potatoes and 1 cup mixed greens with fat-free dressing. Serves 4.

Nutritional Information: 190 calories (38.8% calories from fat); 8g fat; 26g protein; 2g carbohydrate; trace dietary fiber; 92mg cholesterol; 602mg sodium.

HEALTHY SNACK OPTIONS

(**Note:** You will need to add the ingredients for each of these items to the grocery lists.)

- $1/_2$ cup of *Double Oat Granola*: 177 calories (see recipe below)
- 1 *Oat 'n' Honey Granola Bar*: 93 calories (see recipe below)
- 1 cup serving of *Strawberries and Cream:* 115 calories (see recipe below)
- 1 banana with 1 tbsp. almond butter: 207 calories (you can also substitute peanut butter for the almond butter)
- 1 mini-bagel with fat-free cream cheese (2 oz.): 145 calories
- 30 small pretzel sticks: 90 calories
- 2 tbsp. hummus and 1 pita round: 217 calories
- 1 apple with 2 wedges of Laughing Cow® cheese: 151 calories
- 3 cups air-popped popcorn sprinkled with 1 tbsp. parmesan cheese (you can also spray it with nonstick cooking spray and sprinkle with a cajun spice): 120 calories
- 1 cup of *Lemonade* or *Peachy Lemonade:* 15/42 calories (recipes below)
- Snack plate: 25 grapes, 3 tbsp. feta cheese, 6 crackers: 200 calories

SNACK RECIPES

(**Note:** You will need to add the ingredients for each of these items to the grocery lists.)

Double Oat Granola

nonstick cooking spray
$2^1/_2$ cups regular rolled oats
1 cup toasted oat bran cereal
$1/_2$ cup toasted wheat germ
$1/_3$ cup pecans, coarsely chopped
$1/_2$ cup unsweetened applesauce

2 tbsp. honey
1 tbsp. cooking oil
$1/_4$ tsp. ground cinnamon
$1/_3$ cup snipped dried cranberries, snipped dried tart cherries, and/or dried blueberries

Preheat oven to 325°F. Lightly coat a 15 x 10 x 1-inch baking pan with nonstick cooking spray and set aside. In a large bowl, stir together rolled oats, oat bran cereal, wheat germ and pecans. In a separate small bowl, stir together applesauce, honey, cooking oil and cinnamon. Pour applesauce mixture over the cereal mixture and stir using a wooden spoon until the applesauce is evenly distributed. Spread the granola mixture evenly onto the prepared pan and bake about 40 minutes or until golden brown, stirring every 10 minutes. Stir in dried fruit and spread on foil to cool. Store in an airtight container for up to 2 weeks. Makes 5 cups (10 $^1/_2$-cup servings).

Nutritional Information per $^1/_2$ cup serving: 177 calories (29.0% calories from fat); 6g fat; 7g protein; 28g carbohydrate; 5g dietary fiber; 0mg cholesterol; 2mg sodium.

Oat 'n' Honey Granola Bars

nonstick cooking spray
3 cups *Double Oat Granola*
   (see recipe above)
$^1/_2$ cup all-purpose flour
$^1/_4$ cup snipped dried apricots

1 egg
$^1/_3$ cup honey
$^1/_4$ cup cooking oil
$^1/_2$ tsp. apple pie spice

Preheat oven to 325°F. Line an 8 x 8 x 2-inch baking pan with foil and coat lightly with nonstick cooking spray. In a large bowl, combine *Double Oat Granola*, flour and apricots. In a medium bowl, stir together egg, honey, cooking oil and apple pie spice, and then stir into the granola mixture until it is well coated. Press the mixture evenly into the prepared pan. Bake for about 25 minutes or until the granola is lightly browned around the edges. Cool on a wire rack and cut into bars. Makes 24 bars.

Nutritional Information per bar: 93 calories (39% of calories from fat); 4g fat; 2g protein; 13g carbohydrates; 1g dietary fiber; 9mg cholesterol, 11mg sodium.

Strawberries and Cream

1$^1/_2$ cups fat-free sour cream
$^1/_2$ cup brown sugar
$^1/_2$ tbsp. almond extract

1 qt. fresh strawberries, hulled and halved (reserve 6 whole strawberries for the garnish)

Whisk together sour cream, brown sugar and almond extract in a small bowl. In a large bowl, add the halved strawberries and sour cream mixture. Stir gently to mix. Cover and refrigerate until well chilled (about 1 hour). Scoop the strawberries into 6 colorful bowls or chilled sherbet glasses. Garnish with whole strawberries. Serves 6.

Nutritional Information: 115 calories (2.5% calories from fat); trace fat; 5g protein; 25g carbohydrate; 2g dietary fiber; 6mg cholesterol; 49mg sodium.

Lemonade
3 cups cold water
1 cup lemon juice

$^3/_4$ cup sugar substitute
lemon slices

In a 1$^1/_2$-quart pitcher, stir together water, lemon juice and sugar substitute. If desired, chill in the refrigerator. Serve with ice cubes and garnish with lemon slices. Serves 4.

Nutritional Information: 15 calories (0% calories from fat); 0g fat; trace protein; 5g carbohydrate; trace dietary fiber; 0mg cholesterol; 1mg sodium.

Peachy Lemonade
3 cups cold water
1 cup lemon juice
$^3/_4$ cup sugar substitute

lemon slices
1 16-oz. can of peach slices
  (juice pack), chilled and undrained

Prepare *Lemonade* as above. Place half of the can of peach slices in a blender with 1 cup of the *Lemonade*. Cover and blend until smooth and then pour into a large pitcher. Repeat with remaining undrained peaches and 1 cup *Lemonade*. Stir in remaining *Lemonade* and serve over ice. If desired, garnish with peach slices. Serves 4.

Nutritional Information: 42 calories; (1.1% calories from fat); trace fat; 1g protein; 12g carbohydrate; 1g dietary fiber; 0mg cholesterol; 4mg sodium.

DESSERT RECIPES

(**Note:** You will need to add the ingredients for each of these items to the grocery lists.)

Peach Crumble
nonstick cooking spray
8 ripe peaches, peeled,
  pitted and sliced
juice from 1 lemon
$^1/_3$ tsp. ground cinnamon
$^1/_4$ tsp. ground nutmeg

$^1/_2$ cup whole-wheat flour
$^1/_4$ cup packed dark brown sugar
2 tbsp. trans-free margarine,
  cut into thin slices
$^1/_4$ cup quick-cooking oats

Preheat oven to 375°F. Lightly coat a 9-inch pie pan with nonstick cooking spray. Arrange peach slices in the prepared pie pan and sprinkle with lemon juice, cinnamon and nutmeg. In a small bowl, whisk together flour and brown sugar. With your fingers, crumble the margarine into the flour-sugar mixture. Add the oats and stir to mix evenly. Sprinkle the flour mixture on top of the peaches and bake until the peaches are soft and the topping is browned (about 30 minutes). Cut into 8 even slices and serve warm. Serves 8.

Nutritional Information: 116 calories (13.1% calories from fat); 2g fat; 2g protein; 25g carbohydrate; 3g dietary fiber; 0mg cholesterol; 38mg sodium.

Summer Berry Pudding

4 small slices firm white bread,
   crusts removed
1 cup sliced fresh strawberries
1 cup fresh blueberries

1 cup fresh raspberries
2 tbsp. sugar
2 tbsp. water
dash of salt

Place a 1-cup ramekin or similar-size dish on top of a slice of bread and cut around it to trim the bread to fit the dish. Repeat with the remaining 3 slices of bread. Combine the strawberries, blueberries, raspberries, sugar, water and salt in a medium saucepan and cook over medium-high heat until the berries break down (about 5 to 6 minutes). Reserve $1/3$ cup of the mixture for garnish; cover and refrigerate. Place 1 tablespoon of the berry mixture in the bottom of each ramekin and top with a slice of bread. Divide the remaining berry mixture between each, and then top with another slice of bread. Put the puddings on a large plate to catch any overflowing juices. Cover each with plastic wrap, and then place a 15-ounce weight (such as a can of beans) on top of each pudding. Refrigerate for at least 6 hours or up to 2 days. When ready to serve, remove the weight and plastic wrap, run a knife around the inside of the ramekin, and invert onto a dessert plate. Spoon the reserved berry mixture over the puddings. Serves 4.

Nutritional Information: 139 calories (8.4% calories from fat); 1g fat; 3g protein; 30g carbohydrate; 5g dietary fiber; trace cholesterol; 171mg sodium.

Red, White and Blue Berry Parfait

1 8-oz. carton of vanilla lowfat yogurt
$1/4$ tsp. almond extract,
   or $1/2$ tsp. vanilla extract
3 cups fresh blueberries

4 oz. frozen light whipped
   dessert topping, thawed
3 cups fresh raspberries and/or
   cut fresh strawberries

In a large bowl, stir together yogurt and almond extract or vanilla. Fold in whipped topping. Place in 6 12-oz. glasses or dessert dishes, alternating the layers of the berries with the layers of the yogurt mixture. Serves 6.

Nutritional Information: 129 calories (21% of calories from fat); 3g fat (2g saturated fat), 21g carbohydrate; 8g dietary fiber; 2mg cholesterol, 26mg sodium.

Berry Dessert Nachos

$^3/_4$ cup fat-free or light
  dairy sour cream
$^3/_4$ cup frozen light whipped
  dessert topping, thawed
1 tsp. vanilla
$^1/_8$ tsp. ground cinnamon
3 8-inch plain or whole wheat
  flour tortillas

1 tbsp. melted butter
2 tsp. sugar
$^1/_8$ tsp. ground cinnamon
3 cups fresh raspberries
  and/or blackberries
2 tbsp. sliced almonds, toasted
1 tbsp. grated semisweet chocolate

Preheat oven to 400° F. In a small bowl, stir together the sour cream, whipped dessert topping, vanilla and cinnamon. Cover and chill. Lightly brush both sides of each tortilla with melted butter. In a small bowl, stir sugar and cinnamon together and sprinkle over the tortillas. Cut each tortilla into 8 wedges and arrange on two ungreased baking sheets. Bake for 8 to 10 minutes or until crisp. Cool completely. When ready to serve, divide the tortilla wedges among six dessert plates and top with raspberries and/or blackberries and sour cream mixture. Sprinkle with almonds and grated chocolate. Serves 6.

Nutritional Information: 229 calories (33.0% calories from fat); 8g fat; 5g protein; 34g carbohydrate; 6g dietary fiber; 7mg cholesterol; 205mg sodium.

Lemon Cream

$^1/_4$ cup sugar
1 envelope unflavored gelatin
$1^1/_2$ cups water
2 eggs
1 tbsp. finely shredded lemon peel

$^1/_3$ cup lemon juice
4 oz. frozen light whipped
  dessert topping, thawed
lemon peel strips (optional)

Combine the sugar and gelatin in a medium saucepan and stir in water. Cook and stir over medium heat until the mixture bubbles and the gelatin is dissolved. In a separate bowl, beat the the eggs and gradually stir in about half of the gelatin mixture. Return the mixture to the saucepan. Cook over low heat for 2 to 3 minutes or until slightly thickened, stirring constantly. Transfer to a medium bowl and stir in the shredded lemon peel and lemon juice. Chill in ice water for about 20 minutes or just until the mixture thickens slightly, stirring occasionally. Fold the whipped topping into the lemon mixture. Chill again in ice water for about 15 minutes or just until mixture mounds, stirring occasionally. Spoon into individual dessert dishes or soufflé dishes. Cover and chill at least 2 hours or until set. If desired, garnish with lemon peel strips. Makes 6 $1/2$-cup servings.

Nutritional Information: 107 calories (34% of calories from fat); 4g fat (3g saturated fat); 3g protein; 15g carbohydrate; 71mg cholesterol; 37mg sodium.

Berry Pudding Cake

nonstick cooking spray
2 eggs
$1/4$ cup sugar
1 tsp. vanilla
dash of salt
1 cup fat-free milk

$1/2$ cup all-purpose flour
$1/2$ tsp. baking powder
3 cups assorted fresh berries
   (such as raspberries, blueberries,
   and/or sliced strawberries)
powdered sugar (optional)

Preheat oven to 400°F. Lightly coat six 6-ounce individual quiche dishes with nonstick cooking spray. Arrange in a 15 x 10 x 1-inch baking pan and set aside. In a medium bowl, combine eggs, sugar, vanilla and salt. Whisk until light and frothy. Whisk in milk until all ingredients are combined. Add flour and baking powder; whisk until smooth. Divide berries among the prepared quiche dishes and pour the batter over the berries. (Note that the batter will not cover berries completely.) Bake for about 20 minutes or until the cake is puffed and golden brown. Serve warm. If desired, sift powdered sugar over each serving. Serves 6.

Nutritional Information: 134 calories (13.9% calories from fat); 2g fat; 5g protein; 24g carbohydrate; 2g dietary fiber; 71mg cholesterol; 130mg sodium.

Peach-Berry Cobbler

4 cups sliced, peeled fresh peaches,
   or one 16-ounce package frozen
   unsweetened peach slices, thawed

$1/4$ cup cold water
2 tbsp. sugar (or sugar substitute
   equivalent to 2 tbsp. sugar)

4 tsp. cornstarch

1 tbsp. lemon juice

$^1/_4$ tsp. ground allspice,
  cardamom or cinnamon

Biscuit Topping (see recipe below)

2 cups fresh raspberries or frozen
  lightly sweetened raspberries, thawed

In a medium saucepan, combine the peaches, water, sugar (or sugar substitute), cornstarch, lemon juice and allspice (or cardamom or cinnamon). Let stand for 10 minutes. Preheat oven to 400°F. Cook and stir the peach mixture over medium heat until it is thick and bubbly. Stir in the raspberries and heat, stirring gently. Transfer the hot filling to a 2-quart baking dish. Immediately drop the *Biscuit Topping* into small mounds onto the hot filling. Bake for about 20 minutes or until browned and a toothpick inserted into topping comes out clean. Serve warm. Serves 9.

Biscuit Topping

1 cup all-purpose flour

2 tbsp. sugar (or sugar substitute
  equivalent to 2 tbsp. sugar)

$^3/_4$ tsp. baking powder

$^1/_4$ tsp. baking soda

$^1/_8$ tsp. salt

$^1/_4$ tsp. ground allspice,
  cardamom or cinnamon

$^1/_3$ cup plain lowfat yogurt

1 egg, beaten, or $^1/_4$ refrigerated
  or frozen egg product, thawed

2 tbsp. melted butter or margarine

In a medium bowl, combine flour, sugar or sugar substitute, baking powder, baking soda, allspice (or cardamom or cinnamon) and salt. In a small bowl, stir together yogurt, beaten egg (or egg product) and melted butter. Add the egg mixture to the flour mixture, stirring just until moistened.

Nutritional Information: 160 calories (19.6% calories from fat); 4g fat; 3g protein; 30g carbohydrate; 4g dietary fiber; 31mg cholesterol; 146mg sodium.

Pineapple Fresca

3 cups pineapple chunks (if using
  canned pinapple, drain before using)

1 cup water

6 mint leaves

Combine pineapple chunks, water and 6 mint leaves in a blender and process until smooth. Transfer pineapple mixture to a pitcher. Add 2 cups cold water. Serve over ice. Serves 6.

Nutritional Information: 40 calories (2.2% calories from fat); trace fat; 1g protein; 10g carbohydrate; 1g dietary fiber; 0mg cholesterol; 3mg sodium.

Member Survey

Please answer the following questions to help your leader plan your First Place 4 Health meetings so that your needs might be met in this session. Give this form to your leader at the first group meeting.

Name _____ Birth date _____

Please list those who live in your household.

Name	Relationship	Age
_____	_____	___
_____	_____	___
_____	_____	___
_____	_____	___

What church do you attend? _____

Are you interested in receiving more information about our church?

❑ Yes   ❑ No

Occupation _____

What talent or area of expertise would you be willing to share with our class?

_____

Why did you join First Place 4 Health?

_____

With notice, would you be willing to lead a Bible study discussion one week?

❑ Yes   ❑ No

Are you comfortable praying out loud? _____

If the assistant leader were absent, would you be willing to assist in weighing in members and possibly evaluating the Live It Trackers?

❑ Yes   ❑ No

Any other comments:

_____

_____

Personal Weight and Measurement Record

Week	Weight	+ or -	Goal this Session	Pounds to goal
1				
2				
3				
4				
5				
6				

Beginning Measurements

Waist _____ Hips _____ Thighs _____ Chest _____

Ending Measurements

Waist _____ Hips _____ Thighs _____ Chest _____

First Place 4 Health
Prayer Partner

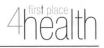

HEALTHY SUMMER
LIVING
Week
2

My soul will rejoice in the LORD
and delight in his salvation.

PSALM 35:9

Date: _____

Name: _____

Home Phone: (_____) _____

Work Phone: (_____) _____

Email: _____

Personal Prayer Concerns:

_____

_____

_____

_____

_____

_____

_____

This form is for prayer requests that are personal to you and your journey in First Place 4 Health. Please complete this form and have it ready to turn in when you arrive at your group meeting.

First Place 4 Health
Prayer Partner

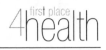

A word aptly spoken is like apples of gold
in settings of silver.

PROVERBS 25:11

Date: _____

Name: _____

Home Phone: (_____) _____

Work Phone: (_____) _____

Email: _____

Personal Prayer Concerns:

_____

_____

_____

_____

_____

_____

_____

This form is for prayer requests that are personal to you and your journey in First Place 4 Health. Please complete this form and have it ready to turn in when you arrive at your group meeting.

First Place 4 Health
Prayer Partner

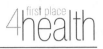

HEALTHY SUMMER
LIVING
Week
6

Whoever gives heed to instruction prospers,
and blessed is he who trusts in the LORD.

PROVERBS 16:20

Date: _____

Name: _____

Home Phone: (_____)_____

Work Phone: (_____)_____

Email: _____

Personal Prayer Concerns:

_____

_____

_____

_____

_____

_____

_____

This form is for prayer requests that are personal to you and your journey in First Place 4 Health. Please complete this form and have it ready to turn in when you arrive at your group meeting.

Live It Tracker

Name: _____ Loss/gain: _____ lbs.

Date: _____ Week #: _____ Calorie Range: _____ My food goal for next week: _____

Activity Level: None, < 30 min/day, 30-60 min/day, 60+ min/day My activity goal for next week:

Group	Daily Calories							
	1300-1400	1500-1600	1700-1800	1900-2000	2100-2200	2300-2400	2500-2600	2700-2800
Fruits	1.5-2 c.	1.5-2 c.	1.5-2 c.	2-2.5 c.	2-2.5 c.	2.5-3.5 c.	3.5-4.5 c.	3.5-4.5 c.
Vegetables	1.5-2 c.	2-2.5 c.	2.5-3 c.	2.5-3 c.	3-3.5 c.	3.5-4.5 c.	4.5-5 c.	4.5-5 c.
Grains	5 oz-eq.	5-6 oz-eq.	6-7 oz-eq.	6-7 oz-eq.	7-8 oz-eq.	8-9 oz-eq.	9-10 oz-eq.	10-11 oz-eq.
Meat & Beans	4 oz-eq.	5 oz-eq.	5-5.5 oz-eq.	5.5-6.5 oz-eq.	6.5-7 oz-eq.	7-7.5 oz-eq.	7-7.5 oz-eq.	7.5-8 oz-eq.
Milk	2-3 c.	3 c.	3 c.	3 c.	3 c.	3 c.	3 c.	3 c.
Healthy Oils	4 tsp.	5 tsp.	5 tsp.	6 tsp.	6 tsp.	7 tsp.	8 tsp.	8 tsp.

Day/Date:

Breakfast: _____ Lunch: _____

Dinner: _____ Snack: _____

Group	Fruits	Vegetables	Grains	Meat & Beans	Milk	Oils
Goal Amount						
Estimate Your Total						
Increase ⇧ or Decrease? ⇩						

Physical Activity: _____ Spiritual Activity: _____

Steps/Miles/Minutes: _____

Day/Date:

Breakfast: _____ Lunch: _____

Dinner: _____ Snack: _____

Group	Fruits	Vegetables	Grains	Meat & Beans	Milk	Oils
Goal Amount						
Estimate Your Total						
Increase ⇧ or Decrease? ⇩						

Physical Activity: _____ Spiritual Activity: _____

Steps/Miles/Minutes: _____

Day/Date:

Breakfast: _____ Lunch: _____

Dinner: _____ Snack: _____

Group	Fruits	Vegetables	Grains	Meat & Beans	Milk	Oils
Goal Amount						
Estimate Your Total						
Increase ⇧ or Decrease? ⇩						

Physical Activity: _____ Spiritual Activity: _____

Steps/Miles/Minutes: _____

Day/Date: ___

Breakfast: _____ Lunch: _____

Dinner: _____ Snack: _____

Group	Fruits	Vegetables	Grains	Meat & Beans	Milk	Oils
Goal Amount						
Estimate Your Total						
Increase ⇧ or Decrease? ⇩						

Physical Activity: _____ Spiritual Activity: _____

Steps/Miles/Minutes: _____ _____

Day/Date: ___

Breakfast: _____ Lunch: _____

Dinner: _____ Snack: _____

Group	Fruits	Vegetables	Grains	Meat & Beans	Milk	Oils
Goal Amount						
Estimate Your Total						
Increase ⇧ or Decrease? ⇩						

Physical Activity: _____ Spiritual Activity: _____

Steps/Miles/Minutes: _____ _____

Day/Date: ___

Breakfast: _____ Lunch: _____

Dinner: _____ Snack: _____

Group	Fruits	Vegetables	Grains	Meat & Beans	Milk	Oils
Goal Amount						
Estimate Your Total						
Increase ⇧ or Decrease? ⇩						

Physical Activity: _____ Spiritual Activity: _____

Steps/Miles/Minutes: _____ _____

Day/Date: ___

Breakfast: _____ Lunch: _____

Dinner: _____ Snack: _____

Group	Fruits	Vegetables	Grains	Meat & Beans	Milk	Oils
Goal Amount						
Estimate Your Total						
Increase ⇧ or Decrease? ⇩						

Physical Activity: _____ Spiritual Activity: _____

Steps/Miles/Minutes: _____ _____

Live It Tracker

Name: _____ Loss/gain: _____ lbs.

Date: _____ Week #: _____ Calorie Range: _____ My food goal for next week: _____

Activity Level: None, < 30 min/day, 30-60 min/day, 60+ min/day My activity goal for next week:

Group	Daily Calories							
	1300-1400	1500-1600	1700-1800	1900-2000	2100-2200	2300-2400	2500-2600	2700-2800
Fruits	1.5-2 c.	1.5-2 c.	1.5-2 c.	2-2.5 c.	2-2.5 c.	2.5-3.5 c.	3.5-4.5 c.	3.5-4.5 c.
Vegetables	1.5-2 c.	2-2.5 c.	2.5-3 c.	2.5-3 c.	3-3.5 c.	3.5-4.5 c.	4.5-5 c.	4.5-5 c.
Grains	5 oz-eq.	5-6 oz-eq.	6-7 oz-eq.	6-7 oz-eq.	7-8 oz-eq.	8-9 oz-eq.	9-10 oz-eq.	10-11 oz-eq.
Meat & Beans	4 oz-eq.	5 oz-eq.	5-5.5 oz-eq.	5.5-6.5 oz-eq.	6.5-7 oz-eq.	7-7.5 oz-eq.	7-7.5 oz-eq.	7.5-8 oz-eq.
Milk	2-3 c.	3 c.	3 c.	3 c.	3 c.	3 c.	3 c.	3 c.
Healthy Oils	4 tsp.	5 tsp.	5 tsp.	6 tsp.	6 tsp.	7 tsp.	8 tsp.	8 tsp.

Day/Date:

Breakfast: _____ Lunch: _____

Dinner: _____ Snack: _____

Group	Fruits	Vegetables	Grains	Meat & Beans	Milk	Oils
Goal Amount						
Estimate Your Total						
Increase ⇧ or Decrease? ⇩						

Physical Activity: _____ Spiritual Activity: _____

Steps/Miles/Minutes: _____

Day/Date:

Breakfast: _____ Lunch: _____

Dinner: _____ Snack: _____

Group	Fruits	Vegetables	Grains	Meat & Beans	Milk	Oils
Goal Amount						
Estimate Your Total						
Increase ⇧ or Decrease? ⇩						

Physical Activity: _____ Spiritual Activity: _____

Steps/Miles/Minutes: _____

Day/Date:

Breakfast: _____ Lunch: _____

Dinner: _____ Snack: _____

Group	Fruits	Vegetables	Grains	Meat & Beans	Milk	Oils
Goal Amount						
Estimate Your Total						
Increase ⇧ or Decrease? ⇩						

Physical Activity: _____ Spiritual Activity: _____

Steps/Miles/Minutes: _____

Day/Date: ____

Breakfast: _____ Lunch: _____

Dinner: _____ Snack: _____

Group	Fruits	Vegetables	Grains	Meat & Beans	Milk	Oils
Goal Amount						
Estimate Your Total						
Increase ⇧ or Decrease? ⇩						

Physical Activity: _____ Spiritual Activity: _____

Steps/Miles/Minutes: _____ _____

Day/Date: ____

Breakfast: _____ Lunch: _____

Dinner: _____ Snack: _____

Group	Fruits	Vegetables	Grains	Meat & Beans	Milk	Oils
Goal Amount						
Estimate Your Total						
Increase ⇧ or Decrease? ⇩						

Physical Activity: _____ Spiritual Activity: _____

Steps/Miles/Minutes: _____ _____

Day/Date: ____

Breakfast: _____ Lunch: _____

Dinner: _____ Snack: _____

Group	Fruits	Vegetables	Grains	Meat & Beans	Milk	Oils
Goal Amount						
Estimate Your Total						
Increase ⇧ or Decrease? ⇩						

Physical Activity: _____ Spiritual Activity: _____

Steps/Miles/Minutes: _____ _____

Day/Date: ____

Breakfast: _____ Lunch: _____

Dinner: _____ Snack: _____

Group	Fruits	Vegetables	Grains	Meat & Beans	Milk	Oils
Goal Amount						
Estimate Your Total						
Increase ⇧ or Decrease? ⇩						

Physical Activity: _____ Spiritual Activity: _____

Steps/Miles/Minutes: _____ _____

Live It Tracker

Name: _____ Loss/gain: _____ lbs.

Date: _____ Week #: _____ Calorie Range: _____ My food goal for next week: _____

Activity Level: None, < 30 min/day, 30-60 min/day, 60+ min/day My activity goal for next week:

Group	Daily Calories							
	1300-1400	1500-1600	1700-1800	1900-2000	2100-2200	2300-2400	2500-2600	2700-2800
Fruits	1.5-2 c.	1.5-2 c.	1.5-2 c.	2-2.5 c.	2-2.5 c.	2.5-3.5 c.	3.5-4.5 c.	3.5-4.5 c.
Vegetables	1.5-2 c.	2-2.5 c.	2.5-3 c.	2.5-3 c.	3-3.5 c.	3.5-4.5 c.	4.5-5 c.	4.5-5 c.
Grains	5 oz-eq.	5-6 oz-eq.	6-7 oz-eq.	6-7 oz-eq.	7-8 oz-eq.	8-9 oz-eq.	9-10 oz-eq.	10-11 oz-eq.
Meat & Beans	4 oz-eq.	5 oz-eq.	5-5.5 oz-eq.	5.5-6.5 oz-eq.	6.5-7 oz-eq.	7-7.5 oz-eq.	7-7.5 oz-eq.	7.5-8 oz-eq.
Milk	2-3 c.	3 c.	3 c.	3 c.	3 c.	3 c.	3 c.	3 c.
Healthy Oils	4 tsp.	5 tsp.	5 tsp.	6 tsp.	6 tsp.	7 tsp.	8 tsp.	8 tsp.

Day/Date:

Breakfast: _____ Lunch: _____

Dinner: _____ Snack: _____

Group	Fruits	Vegetables	Grains	Meat & Beans	Milk	Oils
Goal Amount						
Estimate Your Total						
Increase ⇧ or Decrease? ⇩						

Physical Activity: _____ Spiritual Activity: _____

Steps/Miles/Minutes: _____

Day/Date:

Breakfast: _____ Lunch: _____

Dinner: _____ Snack: _____

Group	Fruits	Vegetables	Grains	Meat & Beans	Milk	Oils
Goal Amount						
Estimate Your Total						
Increase ⇧ or Decrease? ⇩						

Physical Activity: _____ Spiritual Activity: _____

Steps/Miles/Minutes: _____

Day/Date:

Breakfast: _____ Lunch: _____

Dinner: _____ Snack: _____

Group	Fruits	Vegetables	Grains	Meat & Beans	Milk	Oils
Goal Amount						
Estimate Your Total						
Increase ⇧ or Decrease? ⇩						

Physical Activity: _____ Spiritual Activity: _____

Steps/Miles/Minutes: _____

Day/Date:

Breakfast: _____   Lunch: _____

Dinner: _____   Snack: _____

Group	Fruits	Vegetables	Grains	Meat & Beans	Milk	Oils
Goal Amount						
Estimate Your Total						
Increase ⬆ or Decrease? ⬇						

Physical Activity: _____   Spiritual Activity: _____

Steps/Miles/Minutes: _____   _____

Day/Date:

Breakfast: _____   Lunch: _____

Dinner: _____   Snack: _____

Group	Fruits	Vegetables	Grains	Meat & Beans	Milk	Oils
Goal Amount						
Estimate Your Total						
Increase ⬆ or Decrease? ⬇						

Physical Activity: _____   Spiritual Activity: _____

Steps/Miles/Minutes: _____   _____

Day/Date:

Breakfast: _____   Lunch: _____

Dinner: _____   Snack: _____

Group	Fruits	Vegetables	Grains	Meat & Beans	Milk	Oils
Goal Amount						
Estimate Your Total						
Increase ⬆ or Decrease? ⬇						

Physical Activity: _____   Spiritual Activity: _____

Steps/Miles/Minutes: _____   _____

Day/Date:

Breakfast: _____   Lunch: _____

Dinner: _____   Snack: _____

Group	Fruits	Vegetables	Grains	Meat & Beans	Milk	Oils
Goal Amount						
Estimate Your Total						
Increase ⬆ or Decrease? ⬇						

Physical Activity: _____   Spiritual Activity: _____

Steps/Miles/Minutes: _____   _____

Live It Tracker

Name: _____ Loss/gain: _____ lbs.

Date: _____ Week #: ____ Calorie Range: _____ My food goal for next week: _____

Activity Level: None, < 30 min/day, 30-60 min/day, 60+ min/day   My activity goal for next week:

Group	Daily Calories							
	1300-1400	1500-1600	1700-1800	1900-2000	2100-2200	2300-2400	2500-2600	2700-2800
Fruits	1.5-2 c.	1.5-2 c.	1.5-2 c.	2-2.5 c.	2-2.5 c.	2.5-3.5 c.	3.5-4.5 c.	3.5-4.5 c.
Vegetables	1.5-2 c.	2-2.5 c.	2.5-3 c.	2.5-3 c.	3-3.5 c.	3.5-4.5 c.	4.5-5 c.	4.5-5 c.
Grains	5 oz-eq.	5-6 oz-eq.	6-7 oz-eq.	6-7 oz-eq.	7-8 oz-eq.	8-9 oz-eq.	9-10 oz-eq.	10-11 oz-eq.
Meat & Beans	4 oz-eq.	5 oz-eq.	5-5.5 oz-eq.	5.5-6.5 oz-eq.	6.5-7 oz-eq.	7-7.5 oz-eq.	7-7.5 oz-eq.	7.5-8 oz-eq.
Milk	2-3 c.	3 c.	3 c.	3 c.	3 c.	3 c.	3 c.	3 c.
Healthy Oils	4 tsp.	5 tsp.	5 tsp.	6 tsp.	6 tsp.	7 tsp.	8 tsp.	8 tsp.

Day/Date:

Breakfast: _____   Lunch: _____

Dinner: _____   Snack: _____

Group	Fruits	Vegetables	Grains	Meat & Beans	Milk	Oils
Goal Amount						
Estimate Your Total						
Increase ⇧ or Decrease? ⇩						

Physical Activity: _____   Spiritual Activity: _____

Steps/Miles/Minutes: _____

Day/Date:

Breakfast: _____   Lunch: _____

Dinner: _____   Snack: _____

Group	Fruits	Vegetables	Grains	Meat & Beans	Milk	Oils
Goal Amount						
Estimate Your Total						
Increase ⇧ or Decrease? ⇩						

Physical Activity: _____   Spiritual Activity: _____

Steps/Miles/Minutes: _____

Day/Date:

Breakfast: _____   Lunch: _____

Dinner: _____   Snack: _____

Group	Fruits	Vegetables	Grains	Meat & Beans	Milk	Oils
Goal Amount						
Estimate Your Total						
Increase ⇧ or Decrease? ⇩						

Physical Activity: _____   Spiritual Activity: _____

Steps/Miles/Minutes: _____

Day/Date:

Breakfast: _____ Lunch: _____

Dinner: _____ Snack: _____

Group	Fruits	Vegetables	Grains	Meat & Beans	Milk	Oils
Goal Amount						
Estimate Your Total						
Increase ⇧ or Decrease? ⇩						

Physical Activity: _____ Spiritual Activity: _____

Steps/Miles/Minutes: _____ _____

Day/Date:

Breakfast: _____ Lunch: _____

Dinner: _____ Snack: _____

Group	Fruits	Vegetables	Grains	Meat & Beans	Milk	Oils
Goal Amount						
Estimate Your Total						
Increase ⇧ or Decrease? ⇩						

Physical Activity: _____ Spiritual Activity: _____

Steps/Miles/Minutes: _____ _____

Day/Date:

Breakfast: _____ Lunch: _____

Dinner: _____ Snack: _____

Group	Fruits	Vegetables	Grains	Meat & Beans	Milk	Oils
Goal Amount						
Estimate Your Total						
Increase ⇧ or Decrease? ⇩						

Physical Activity: _____ Spiritual Activity: _____

Steps/Miles/Minutes: _____ _____

Day/Date:

Breakfast: _____ Lunch: _____

Dinner: _____ Snack: _____

Group	Fruits	Vegetables	Grains	Meat & Beans	Milk	Oils
Goal Amount						
Estimate Your Total						
Increase ⇧ or Decrease? ⇩						

Physical Activity: _____ Spiritual Activity: _____

Steps/Miles/Minutes: _____ _____

Live It Tracker

Name: _____ Loss/gain: _____ lbs.

Date: _____ Week #: _____ Calorie Range: _____ My food goal for next week: _____

Activity Level: None, < 30 min/day, 30-60 min/day, 60+ min/day   My activity goal for next week:

Group	Daily Calories							
	1300-1400	1500-1600	1700-1800	1900-2000	2100-2200	2300-2400	2500-2600	2700-2800
Fruits	1.5-2 c.	1.5-2 c.	1.5-2 c.	2-2.5 c.	2-2.5 c.	2.5-3.5 c.	3.5-4.5 c.	3.5-4.5 c.
Vegetables	1.5-2 c.	2-2.5 c.	2.5-3 c.	2.5-3 c.	3-3.5 c.	3.5-4.5 c.	4.5-5 c.	4.5-5 c.
Grains	5 oz-eq.	5-6 oz-eq.	6-7 oz-eq.	6-7 oz-eq.	7-8 oz-eq.	8-9 oz-eq.	9-10 oz-eq.	10-11 oz-eq.
Meat & Beans	4 oz-eq.	5 oz-eq.	5-5.5 oz-eq.	5.5-6.5 oz-eq.	6.5-7 oz-eq.	7-7.5 oz-eq.	7-7.5 oz-eq.	7.5-8 oz-eq.
Milk	2-3 c.	3 c.	3 c.	3 c.	3 c.	3 c.	3 c.	3 c.
Healthy Oils	4 tsp.	5 tsp.	5 tsp.	6 tsp.	6 tsp.	7 tsp.	8 tsp.	8 tsp.

Day/Date:

Breakfast: _____   Lunch: _____

Dinner: _____   Snack: _____

Group	Fruits	Vegetables	Grains	Meat & Beans	Milk	Oils
Goal Amount						
Estimate Your Total						
Increase ⇧ or Decrease? ⇩						

Physical Activity: _____   Spiritual Activity: _____

Steps/Miles/Minutes: _____

Day/Date:

Breakfast: _____   Lunch: _____

Dinner: _____   Snack: _____

Group	Fruits	Vegetables	Grains	Meat & Beans	Milk	Oils
Goal Amount						
Estimate Your Total						
Increase ⇧ or Decrease? ⇩						

Physical Activity: _____   Spiritual Activity: _____

Steps/Miles/Minutes: _____

Day/Date:

Breakfast: _____   Lunch: _____

Dinner: _____   Snack: _____

Group	Fruits	Vegetables	Grains	Meat & Beans	Milk	Oils
Goal Amount						
Estimate Your Total						
Increase ⇧ or Decrease? ⇩						

Physical Activity: _____   Spiritual Activity: _____

Steps/Miles/Minutes: _____

Day/Date:

Breakfast: _____ Lunch: _____

Dinner: _____ Snack: _____

Group	Fruits	Vegetables	Grains	Meat & Beans	Milk	Oils
Goal Amount						
Estimate Your Total						
Increase ⇧ or Decrease? ⇩						

Physical Activity: _____ Spiritual Activity: _____

Steps/Miles/Minutes: _____

Day/Date:

Breakfast: _____ Lunch: _____

Dinner: _____ Snack: _____

Group	Fruits	Vegetables	Grains	Meat & Beans	Milk	Oils
Goal Amount						
Estimate Your Total						
Increase ⇧ or Decrease? ⇩						

Physical Activity: _____ Spiritual Activity: _____

Steps/Miles/Minutes: _____

Day/Date:

Breakfast: _____ Lunch: _____

Dinner: _____ Snack: _____

Group	Fruits	Vegetables	Grains	Meat & Beans	Milk	Oils
Goal Amount						
Estimate Your Total						
Increase ⇧ or Decrease? ⇩						

Physical Activity: _____ Spiritual Activity: _____

Steps/Miles/Minutes: _____

Day/Date:

Breakfast: _____ Lunch: _____

Dinner: _____ Snack: _____

Group	Fruits	Vegetables	Grains	Meat & Beans	Milk	Oils
Goal Amount						
Estimate Your Total						
Increase ⇧ or Decrease? ⇩						

Physical Activity: _____ Spiritual Activity: _____

Steps/Miles/Minutes: _____

Live It Tracker

Name: _____ Loss/gain: _____ lbs.

Date: _____ Week #: _____ Calorie Range: _____ My food goal for next week: _____

Activity Level: None, < 30 min/day, 30-60 min/day, 60+ min/day My activity goal for next week:

Group	Daily Calories							
	1300-1400	1500-1600	1700-1800	1900-2000	2100-2200	2300-2400	2500-2600	2700-2800
Fruits	1.5-2 c.	1.5-2 c.	1.5-2 c.	2-2.5 c.	2-2.5 c.	2.5-3.5 c.	3.5-4.5 c.	3.5-4.5 c.
Vegetables	1.5-2 c.	2-2.5 c.	2.5-3 c.	2.5-3 c.	3-3.5 c.	3.5-4.5 c.	4.5-5 c.	4.5-5 c.
Grains	5 oz-eq.	5-6 oz-eq.	6-7 oz-eq.	6-7 oz-eq.	7-8 oz-eq.	8-9 oz-eq.	9-10 oz-eq.	10-11 oz-eq.
Meat & Beans	4 oz-eq.	5 oz-eq.	5-5.5 oz-eq.	5.5-6.5 oz-eq.	6.5-7 oz-eq.	7-7.5 oz-eq.	7-7.5 oz-eq.	7.5-8 oz-eq.
Milk	2-3 c.	3 c.	3 c.	3 c.	3 c.	3 c.	3 c.	3 c.
Healthy Oils	4 tsp.	5 tsp.	5 tsp.	6 tsp.	6 tsp.	7 tsp.	8 tsp.	8 tsp.

Day/Date:

Breakfast: _____ Lunch: _____

Dinner: _____ Snack: _____

Group	Fruits	Vegetables	Grains	Meat & Beans	Milk	Oils
Goal Amount						
Estimate Your Total						
Increase ⇧ or Decrease? ⇩						

Physical Activity: _____ Spiritual Activity: _____

Steps/Miles/Minutes: _____

Day/Date:

Breakfast: _____ Lunch: _____

Dinner: _____ Snack: _____

Group	Fruits	Vegetables	Grains	Meat & Beans	Milk	Oils
Goal Amount						
Estimate Your Total						
Increase ⇧ or Decrease? ⇩						

Physical Activity: _____ Spiritual Activity: _____

Steps/Miles/Minutes: _____

Day/Date:

Breakfast: _____ Lunch: _____

Dinner: _____ Snack: _____

Group	Fruits	Vegetables	Grains	Meat & Beans	Milk	Oils
Goal Amount						
Estimate Your Total						
Increase ⇧ or Decrease? ⇩						

Physical Activity: _____ Spiritual Activity: _____

Steps/Miles/Minutes: _____

Day/Date:

Breakfast: _____   Lunch: _____

Dinner: _____   Snack: _____

Group	Fruits	Vegetables	Grains	Meat & Beans	Milk	Oils
Goal Amount						
Estimate Your Total						
Increase ⇧ or Decrease? ⇩						

Physical Activity: _____   Spiritual Activity: _____

Steps/Miles/Minutes: _____

Day/Date:

Breakfast: _____   Lunch: _____

Dinner: _____   Snack: _____

Group	Fruits	Vegetables	Grains	Meat & Beans	Milk	Oils
Goal Amount						
Estimate Your Total						
Increase ⇧ or Decrease? ⇩						

Physical Activity: _____   Spiritual Activity: _____

Steps/Miles/Minutes: _____

Day/Date:

Breakfast: _____   Lunch: _____

Dinner: _____   Snack: _____

Group	Fruits	Vegetables	Grains	Meat & Beans	Milk	Oils
Goal Amount						
Estimate Your Total						
Increase ⇧ or Decrease? ⇩						

Physical Activity: _____   Spiritual Activity: _____

Steps/Miles/Minutes: _____

Day/Date:

Breakfast: _____   Lunch: _____

Dinner: _____   Snack: _____

Group	Fruits	Vegetables	Grains	Meat & Beans	Milk	Oils
Goal Amount						
Estimate Your Total						
Increase ⇧ or Decrease? ⇩						

Physical Activity: _____   Spiritual Activity: _____

Steps/Miles/Minutes: _____